How to be a
Healthy
VEGAN

Your Ultimate Plant-Based
Nutrition Guide

By Caroline Trickey APD
Clinical Dietitian and Culinary Nutritionist

Disclaimer

Please note that the advice in this book is for general purposes only and is intended to help you understand vegan eating. The publisher and author accept no liability for damages arising from information in this book. For more tailored advice on nutritional requirements during pregnancy and breastfeeding, childhood development, sporting requirements and other special dietary considerations, please consult an accredited practicing dietitian (APD) who specialises in plant-based eating for advice specific to your individual needs.

NATIONAL LIBRARY OF AUSTRALIA

A catalogue record for this book is available from the National Library of Australia

ISBN 978-0-6481700-1-3

Cover, index and internal design by Puddingburn Publishing Services

Define: "Vegan"

Someone whose nutritional intake comes entirely from plants

Quick vegan overview

VEGAN DIETS INCLUDE:

- ✔ Fruit and vegetables
- ✔ Legumes (e.g. lentils, split peas, chickpeas, dried beans)
- ✔ Soy foods (e.g. tofu, tempeh and soymilk)
- ✔ Nuts and seeds
- ✔ Breads, cereals and grains

VEGAN DIETS EXCLUDE:

- ✘ Meat, poultry, fish and seafood
- ✘ Dairy products
- ✘ Eggs
- ✘ Honey, gelatine and other animal-derived ingredients or food additives
- ✘ Vegans avoid leather, wool, silk, cosmetics, soaps and shampoos with ingredients derived from animal products or tested on animals

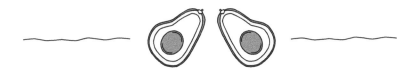

Contents

Introduction

A well-planned vegan intake is healthy, nutritionally adequate and able to provide health benefits in the prevention and treatment of certain illnesses. Appropriately planned and balanced vegan intakes are also suitable during any stage of life, including pregnancy, breastfeeding, infancy, childhood, adolescence, as we age and for athletes.

There are many reasons for the increasing interest in wanting to be vegan, including moral and ethical considerations such as animal welfare, environmental concerns and a desire for overall improved health. However, becoming vegan is not a decision to make lightly. Despite it possibly being the healthiest way to eat for us and our planet, eating a well-balanced vegan intake that provides all the nutrients your body needs to survive and thrive requires a great deal of attention, knowledge, planning, preparation and execution. With that in mind, I have written this book to help you do exactly that more easily.

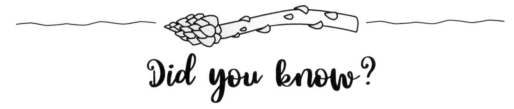

Did you know?

A healthy, well balanced vegan intake tends to be lower in saturated fat, devoid of cholesterol and has higher levels of dietary fibre, magnesium and potassium, vitamins C and E, folate, carotenoids, flavonoids and other health-benefiting phytonutrients.
This may explain some of the health advantages of being vegan, which includes preventing, treating or reversing:

- ❖ Heart disease
- ❖ High blood pressure
- ❖ Type 2 diabetes
- ❖ Digestive problems
- ❖ Constipation and bowel problems

It may also provide beneficial results in the treatment of certain cancers and kidney disease. Furthermore, due to the high fibre content of plant foods, a vegan intake may assist with weight management.

As an adult, how you choose to eat is very much your own personal choice and should be of no consequence to anyone else (despite the tendency for others to comment on it). However, it is your responsibility to obtain an overall healthy balance.

I have recently heard the term "vegan-ish" whereby a person eats purely vegan at home, but when eating out or at friends' places may opt for vegetarian choices. By all means, your eating style doesn't have to fit perfectly into a box. You absolutely get to choose what you eat. Having said that however, this book is directed at those wanting to follow a purely vegan intake as it will explain how to obtain all the nutrients your body needs.

Nutritional deficiencies are a concern for everyone

The average Australian (who isn't vegan) doesn't eat the recommended daily amount of vegetables or fruit. These foods provide vitally important nutrients for optimal health, so everyone is susceptible to nutritional deficiencies. However, excluding many readily available foods obviously can increase your risk if you don't understand, pay attention and take the necessary actions to make sure you get what your body needs.

Nutrients that vegans need to pay particular attention to include protein, omega-3 fatty acids, iron, calcium, zinc and vitamin B12. A vegan diet can meet current recommendations for all nutrients except vitamin D, which comes mainly from sunlight and vitamin B12, which is only naturally present in animal foods. I will discuss that in more detail soon. Meanwhile, on the following page is an easy table of reference outlining the major nutrients your body requires and vegan sources.

Easy vegan swaps

Food	Major nutrients	Vegan alternative	Health benefits
Meat: • Chicken • Lamb • Pork • Veal • Kangaroo	Protein, iron and zinc	Legumes (lentils, beans, chickpeas), soybeans and soy products (tofu, tempeh, milk) Nuts and seeds Pumpkin seeds, Cashews	Minimal saturated fat High in fibre Sources of important phytonutrients
Fish	Omega-3 fats and protein	Walnuts Linseeds, chia seeds Flaxseed oil	Environmentally friendly Free of mercury and other toxins
Eggs	Protein	Ground linseeds or chia seeds Tofu	Good sources of ALA omega-3 fatty acid Cholesterol free Minimal saturated fat
Dairy • Milk • Cheese • Yoghurt	Protein and calcium	Plant-based milks: nut milks (e.g. almond), soy, coconut milk, oat milk, rice milk (high GI) Nut cheese Soy or coconut yoghurt Tahini Almonds	Calcium is just as easily absorbed from soy milk and better absorbed from (low oxalate) green vegetables than dairy Green vegetables also contain other nutrients important for bone health
	Calcium	Dried figs Leafy greens such as kale, broccoli and Asian greens	
Honey	Carbohydrate	Maple syrup Agave nectar Rice malt syrup Golden syrup Cane sugar	All sweeteners are roughly equal when it comes to health
	Carbohydrate	Blackstrap molasses	Good source of both iron and calcium
Gelatine	None (used as a thickener)	Agar agar	Contains iron and magnesium

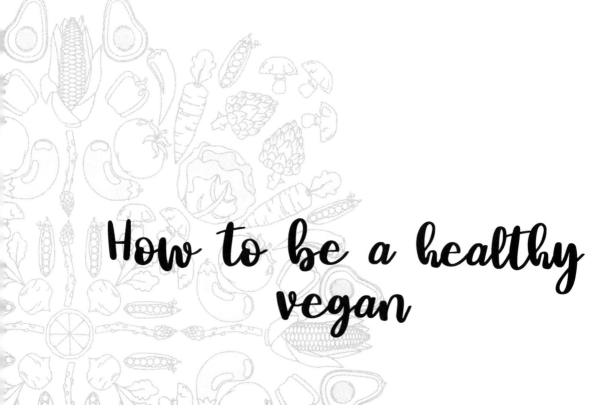

How to be a healthy vegan

Food is vital for life. At its most basic it provides the energy and nutrients we need to survive. The human body requires a regular intake of food to develop, grow, move, work, play, think and learn as well as heal and repair.

Food also brings us together. It is important socially, being the central feature at most social gatherings. We use it to help us celebrate and commiserate—from birthdays, weddings and other special occasions like Christmas to funerals, and here in Australia we have whole festivals focused on celebrating food. So, it is important when choosing to eat differently from others that you take on the responsibility to plan appropriately around these times to ensure you continue to maintain an adequate intake while taking part in social interactions. Also be aware that while many restaurants in most capital cities in Australia now cater for vegans, you may not find the same considerations while travelling around the countryside or overseas.

WHAT IS A WELL BALANCED INTAKE?

All food is made up of the same essential components or nutrients. These include the macronutrients (protein, carbohydrate and fat) as well as the micronutrients (vitamins and minerals). All food differs in quantity and amounts of the nutrients it contains. Your body requires a variety of these nutrients, in the correct quantities from the food you eat, to stay in peak health.

While cola, potato chips and certain donuts may qualify as 'vegan', common sense tells you that those foods are not healthy. It's important to understand the difference between a vegan intake and a properly balanced vegan intake. Following a vegan way of eating requires a fair bit of focus to get a healthy amount of all the vital nutrients your body needs for optimal function. Obviously, the most focus is required when first making the shift to veganism, but it's important you also do not become complacent over time as if you do, your health may suffer.

The consequences of not achieving a well-balanced intake could result in slower healing and repair, lethargy, tiredness and inability to concentrate as well as increased susceptibility to illnesses and disease.

Top tips for getting all the nutrients you need:

❖ Know your nutrients and the best food sources
❖ Have a well-stocked pantry
❖ Plan your intake to give yourself the best chance to achieve a good variety and the correct amounts of nutrients
❖ Have a collection of at least 5 super-quick and easy meals that take under 10 minutes to prepare and keep the ingredients on hand (further information on how to do this is found later in this book)
❖ Have your kitchen set up to streamline the cooking process
❖ Prepare and cook in batches
❖ Take food with you to work, or when away from home for long periods of time
❖ Know where you can access healthy vegan meals and/or snacks as a back-up when out and about
❖ Take a vitamin B12 supplement daily

If in doubt, get blood tests to monitor levels of important nutrients like iron and vitamin B12

Notes

_____

_____

_____

_____

_____

_____

_____

_____

_____

_____

_____

_____

_____

_____

_____

_____

Understanding your macronutrients

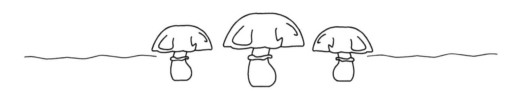

Protein, carbohydrate and fat are macronutrients —
the main components of your intake that your body
requires in relatively large amounts for normal function
and good health.

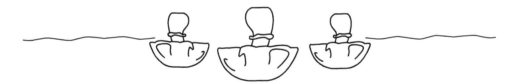

PROTEIN

Protein has both structural and functional properties. It is the building block of the 50 trillion cells from which your body is made. Protein maintains muscles, bone, cartilage, organs, skin, blood and immune cells. It is also used to make hormones, enzymes and neurotransmitters. Getting enough protein helps your muscles repair after exercise, supports your immune system to fight infections and heal wounds, and maintains healthy hair, skin and nails. The protein in your body is continually breaking down and resynthesised in a process called 'protein turnover', and since protein cannot be stored in the body, it important to meet your daily protein needs.

Proteins are made from long chains of amino acids that your body breaks down during digestion. After being digested, these amino acids are absorbed, put back together and used to make new proteins such as brain cells, muscle tissue, hormones, enzymes and immune cells.

There are about 20 different amino acids commonly used by your body. The human body can make some amino acids; however, there are nine amino acids, known as 'essential' amino acids (EAAs), which must come from the food you eat because they cannot be made by your body. Adults require eight EAAs: leucine, isoleucine, valine, threonine, methionine, phenylalanine, tryptophan and lysine. Children also need histidine, which is an essential ninth amino acid.

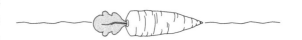

Many people think that a high-protein intake leads to increased muscle mass. This is not true. It is the stimulation of muscle tissue through exercise, not extra dietary protein, which leads to muscle growth.

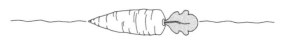

PROTEIN

REQUIREMENTS

How much protein you need each day depends on your body weight, age, health and your activity levels. For most vegans, a protein intake of 0.9 grams per kilogram of body weight will meet your daily needs. So, for example, if you weigh 60 kg, you need 54 grams of protein a day. Or for ease of calculation you may prefer to just use 1.0 gram per kilogram of body weight.

For adults over 70, to help preserve muscle mass and function, the intake suggested is 1.0–1.2 grams of protein per kilogram of body weight per day. This intake is also suggested for those doing a lot of exercise, when pregnant or breastfeeding as well as certain other times when the body makes new tissue, for example, post-surgery or trauma.

You can certainly get all your protein needs from plant-based foods. In fact, if you think about it, the protein in animals originated from plants as cows and sheep are essentially vegan! All you need to do is make sure you eat a variety of plant foods over the course of a day and meet your energy needs. You may like to plan your intake accordingly and I have included information on how to do this towards the end of the book.

Plant foods that contain the most protein include lentils, split peas, chickpeas, dried beans, soybeans, tofu and other products made from soy, as well as nuts and seeds. Note that there are smaller amounts of protein in wholegrains, for example most wholegrain bread is around 10 per cent protein and even fruit and vegetables contain a little protein, for example, bananas contain about 2 per cent protein while mushrooms and kale have around 3 per cent.

Including protein-rich plant foods in all meals can help you meet your daily recommended intake. If you include snacks, you may like to consider protein in those too. Eating protein-rich food can help to fill you up and keep you feeling full for longer.

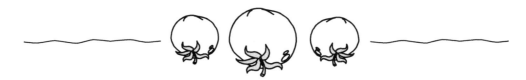

Did you know?

Although carbohydrates are the body's preferred fuel source, about 10 per cent of energy is obtained from protein.

A very high protein intake in excess of your body's needs can cause the build-up of ammonia, a protein metabolism by-product. In high levels, ammonia is extremely dangerous to the body. It is converted into urea by the kidneys and eliminated from the body in your urine. The more protein you eat each day, the more work your kidneys must do to get rid of the ammonia. However, vegan diets typically have a better balance between carbohydrate and protein, so this is only an issue when eating a meat-based diet.

WHAT IS PROTEIN COMBINING?

Protein-rich animal foods contain large amounts of all the EAAs required by your body in a balanced quantity and are referred to as 'complete' proteins.

Protein rich plant foods contain all the EAAs you require but the amounts of one or two of these amino acids may be low. For example, legumes are low in an amino acid called methionine and many grains are low in lysine.

Different plant foods are low in different amino acids but when combined they make a complete set (complementary proteins). It was once thought that certain combinations of plant foods, such as legumes with grains, had to be eaten at the same meal for you to get all the EAAs. We now know that the body keeps a daily pool of these indispensable amino acids in fluids between cells and in the intestine, which can be used to complement dietary proteins so protein combining is not necessary at mealtimes. Simply eating a wide variety of plant-based protein over the day, that is, grains plus legumes plus nuts and seeds, ensures your protein needs will be easily met. Eating this way will also provide you with an adequate intake of energy and all other nutrients, including iron, zinc, calcium and vitamin B12*, which are required for optimal health.

*Note: Vitamin B12 is usually found in animal products such as eggs, dairy and meat. However, it is often added to nutritional yeast and in fortified soy products and fortified soy and some other plant milks. Always check labels.

A few plant-based foods are actually 'complete' proteins. They are soy, quinoa and amaranth.

14

PROTEIN-RICH PLANT FOODS

Legumes, lentils, split peas, beans and chickpeas

Also called pulses, legumes are the seeds from plants whose fruit is enclosed in a pod.

As well as being protein 'powerhouses', legumes are the richest plant source of iron, zinc, other trace minerals and fibre. They are also high in many phytonutrients with antioxidant and anti-cancer properties such as isoflavones, phenolic acids, tannins and phytates.

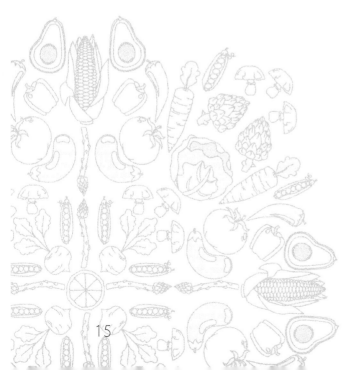

When it comes to nutrition, it's hard to beat legumes as they are one of the most nutritious foods available. Legumes are:

- ❖ A valuable source of protein. Half a cup of cooked legumes contains around 7 grams of protein
- ❖ High in fibre to maintain digestive and bowel health and reduce your risk of bowel cancer. Half a cup of cooked legumes contains between 4 and 7 grams of fibre. You need more than 30 grams a day
- ❖ A good source of soluble fibre which can help lower LDL cholesterol levels and reduce your cardiovascular disease risk
- ❖ A low-GI source of carbohydrate. This means that legumes will keep you full for a good length of time and provide a sustainable source of energy. They are also an excellent food to help prevent and manage diabetes
- ❖ An important source of B-group vitamins, which are your 'energy vitamins', including folate, an essential requirement for everyone, but especially important during pregnancy
- ❖ A source of the minerals iron, zinc, magnesium and calcium
- ❖ An excellent source of phytonutrients (with powerful antioxidant and other health-benefiting effects)
- ❖ A very small but relevant source of essential omega-3 fatty acids
- ❖ Low in saturated fat
- ❖ Low in calories/kilojoules

LENTILS

Lentils are the easiest of all the legumes to cook as they do not require soaking, unlike dried beans and chickpeas, and they are quick to cook as they are done in 8 to 20 minutes. Plus, they are quite bland so absorb the flavour of the foods they are cooked in, from stock to soups, curries and casseroles.

In Australia we have access to four different types of lentils:

❖ Red lentils, which are usually split
❖ Brown/green lentils
❖ Puy or French/ Australian green lentils
❖ Black Beluga lentils

RED LENTILS

Red lentils are the most common type of lentil and are sold predominantly as split lentils. They are a salmon-pink colour when dry but turn golden when cooked. These lentils are very mild in flavour, so they tend to take on the flavour of the foods with which they are cooked. Since they cook within 8 to 10 minutes, they are the fastest to cook of all the lentils. Best in purées, dips, patties or soups as they are quite mushy when cooked. They are also a great gluten-free, high-fibre way to thicken gravies, stews, casseroles and curries.

BROWN/ GREEN LENTILS

These are the only type of lentils you can currently buy pre-cooked in tins but are also easy to find in dry form. They take around 20 minutes to cook and have a slight earthy flavour which I enjoy.

PUY LENTILS, FRENCH OR AUSTRALIAN GREEN LENTILS

Small slate-green lentils, delicate with a slightly peppery flavour, Puy lentils retain their shape when cooked. They only take around 20 minutes to cook. They make a delicious side dish, prepared simply with just olive oil, fresh parsley or thyme, salt and pepper. Their name comes from the Le Puy region in France where they were originally grown. They are now also grown in Australia. The Australian-grown variety is called the French or Australian green lentil.

BLACK BELUGA LENTILS

These are one of the smallest in the lentil family. Shiny black in colour, they are super-easy to cook, taking only 15 to 20 minutes of boiling. They look like caviar (hence the name), so make an interesting garnish on top of canapés. They're also great in soups and salads.

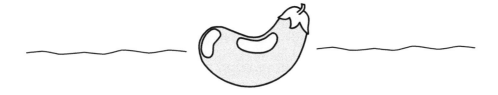

How to cook dried lentils

1. Rinse first then place in a large pot and cover with at least three times the volume of water.
2. Place a lid on the pot and bring to the boil over high heat.
3. Turn heat down to a simmer and cook, half covered for 10 to 20 minutes, depending on the type of lentil, age and how well you like them cooked.

NOTE: DO NOT ADD SALT WHEN COOKING LENTILS BECAUSE THIS SLOWS DOWN THE COOKING PROCESS.

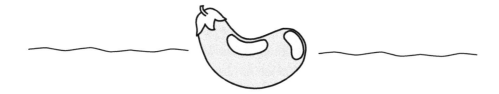

SPLIT PEAS

Split peas could easily be mistaken for lentils as they look very similar. However, they come from a different species of plant. They are also different from fresh garden peas, which are in season in spring and available all year round frozen.

'Field peas', as this variety of split peas is called, are grown specifically to be dried as they are too tough to be eaten fresh. After harvesting, they are podded, skinned and dried, and then usually split either naturally or mechanically. The splitting process increases the surface area, so reduces cooking time.

Available in yellow or green, split peas are probably most well-known as a main ingredient in pea (and ham) soup, where either colour can be used. The yellow ones, sometimes called chana dhal (dal), are used to make dhal and fava dip in Greece. The two colours are the same nutritionally, but green peas are slightly sweeter than the yellow, milder flavoured ones.

Like lentils, they do not need to be soaked before cooking. However, as they take a lot longer to cook than lentils (approx. 50 minutes), many people prefer to pre-soak them to cut down the cooking time.

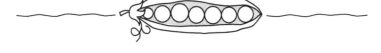

How to cook split peas

1. Place in a colander and rinse, then transfer to a large saucepan and cover with at least triple the amount of cold water. Place a lid on the pot and bring to the boil over high heat.
2. Turn heat down to a simmer and cook, half covered for 50 to 60 minutes.
3. Pre-soaked peas (soaked overnight) will take 30 to 40 minutes to cook.
4. In a pressure cooker, split peas will take about 15 minutes and pre-soaked peas take about 10 minutes.

NOTE: DO NOT ADD SALT WHEN COOKING SPLIT PEAS BECAUSE THIS SLOWS DOWN THE COOKING PROCESS.

CHICKPEAS

I love the spherical shape of chickpeas, their firm but soft texture and mild flavour which lend themselves to all sorts of interesting dishes and cuisines. In tinned form, they are my go-to legume when I am in a hurry.

Chickpeas are an amazingly versatile addition to a wide variety of dishes; everything from soups, dips and salads to curries and tagines. They are also the main ingredient in falafels, the deliciously tasty Lebanese deep-fried balls.

Besan flour, which is made by grinding chickpeas, can be used in baked goods, vegetablefritters and makes a great flatbread which can be used as a pizza base.

How to cook chickpeas

- ❖ Chickpeas are sold pre-cooked in tins or in dried form.
- ❖ Tinned chickpeas are very convenient and only require draining then rinsing under cool running water before use. If used to make a dip or in a salad, they don't need to be heated, but sometimes I like to 'toast' them in a pan with some olive oil and spices. For other recipes such as soups or stews, add them at the end and cook just long enough to heat them through (2 to 3 minutes).
- ❖ Dried chickpeas need to be soaked overnight and then cooked so that they soften up. Home-cooked chickpeas are more flavoursome than tinned, come at a fraction of the cost, and can be cooked to your desired texture such as firm or soft. Don't throw out the cooking water (called aquafaba) as it can be used in baking and to make mayonnaise.
- ❖ One cup of dry chickpeas yields three cups when cooked, which is equal to a little more than two 400 gram tins.
- ❖ Tinned chickpeas are a great pantry staple. They can be stored indefinitely if kept cool. Dried chickpeas should be stored in an air-tight container at cool room temperature. It is best to use them within 6 months because as they get older, they take longer to cook.
- ❖ Leftover cooked chickpeas will keep for 3 to 4 days in the refrigerator, stored in an air-tight container. They can also be frozen.

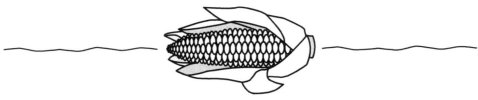

How to cook dried chickpeas

- ❖ Place the chickpeas in a large bowl. Cover with at least triple the amount of cold water. Cover bowl and set aside overnight to soak.
- ❖ The next day, drain well, rinse then transfer to a saucepan or large pot. Cover with fresh water, bring to the boil, then reduce heat to a simmer and cook until tender, approximately 40 minutes to one hour. Alternatively, you can cook them using a pressure cooker (after a pre-soak overnight) and they take about 18 minutes.

NOTE: DO NOT ADD SALT WHEN COOKING CHICKPEAS BECAUSE THIS SLOWS DOWN THE COOKING PROCESS.

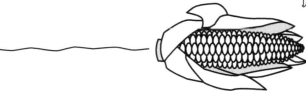

VARIETIES OF CHICKPEAS

There are two main types of chickpeas—Desi and Kabuli, distinguished mainly by seed size, shape and colour.

Desi are smaller and vary in colour from brown, light brown, fawn, yellow, orange, black or green. They are normally de-hulled and split to make dhal and are popular in India. My local Indian grocery stocks the whole brown desi chickpeas which I love to use.

Kabuli are larger. They are white to cream in colour and are almost exclusively used whole. They are preferred throughout the Mediterranean region and the ones most readily available in Australia.

BEANS

There are so many different varieties of beans, from adzuki to kidney to mung, with all their glorious colours and shapes. Most come either pre-cooked in tins or are available in dried form.

Tinned beans are already cooked so they only need to be drained and rinsed before use. This also removes most of the salt if they are tinned in salted water.

Dried beans, except adzuki, black eyed peas and mung beans, need to be soaked overnight before you cook them.

You can cook beans on the stove in a pot, but I prefer to use a pressure cooker as it is much faster. If you are going to cook beans regularly, I highly recommend investing in a good pressure cooker.

How to cook dried beans

Start by soaking them. Combine with at least triple the amount of cold water, cover and set aside overnight (at least 8 hours). The next day, drain well, rinse then transfer to a large pot or pressure cooker.

IN A POT:

- ❖ Put the pre-soaked and drained beans into your pot and cover with cold water. Don't salt the water as this makes the beans tough. Place a lid on the pot and bring to the boil. Skim off any sediment as it rises to the surface.
- ❖ When at a boil, turn heat down, partially cover with lid and cook beans until tender, topping up with boiling water from the kettle as needed. When cooked, drain.
- ❖ Refer to Legume Cooking Guide on the following page for cooking times. Note that cooking times do vary and older beans take longer to cook.

IN A PRESSURE COOKER:

- ❖ Drain soaked beans, put in pressure cooker and just cover with water. Place lid on securely and bring up to pressure with high heat, then turn heat down to simmer for the time listed in the Legume Cooking Guide on the following page.
- ❖ Note that natural release allows the pressure cooker to come down to room temperature naturally. Fast release is when you place the hot, sealed pressure cooker under cold water to cool it down faster.
- ❖ If you do not have time to soak beans overnight, try my alternate 'quick soak' method:
- ❖ Bring a large pot of water to the boil, add beans, and allow the water to return to boiling.
- ❖ Turn off heat, cover and stand for one hour, then drain, rinse and cook for time as listed in the Legume Cooking Guide.

Legume Culinary Guide

Legume	Culinary suggestions
Adzuki beans, also known as aduki, field peas or red beans	Burgers, soups, stews, sweet bean paste, Japanese and Chinese dishes
Black beans, also known as turtle beans	Burgers, soups, stews or casseroles, rice dishes and Latin American dishes, chocolate cake and brownies
Black-eyed peas, also known as cowpeas	Salads, soups, casseroles and Southern dishes
Borlotti beans, also known as cranberry or Roman beans	Soups (especially minestrone), salads and casseroles
Cannellini beans	Dips, burgers, salads, soups, casseroles, pasta dishes, cakes
Chickpeas, also known as garbanzo beans	Hummus, burgers or falafel, salads, soups, casseroles, Spanish and Indian dishes
Edamame, also known as green soybeans	Snack, dips, salads, stir fries, casseroles and rice dishes
Fava beans, also known as broad beans	Dips, falafels, stews and side dishes
Lentils	Dips, salads, burgers, casseroles, stews, side dishes, dhal and other Indian dishes
Lima beans, also known as butter or Madagascar beans	Dips, salads, soups, casseroles, cakes
Mung beans	Sprouted (bean sprouts), soups, dhal, casseroles
Red kidney beans	Dips, salads (especially as part of 4 or 5-bean mix), soups, stews or casseroles, chilli and rice dishes
Roasted soy beans or roasted chickpeas/'chic-nuts'	Snack or garnish for soups and salads
Split peas	Soups, dhal, fava dip

Legume Cooking Guide

Legume	Soak overnight	Cook on stove	Cook in pressure cooker—natural release	Cook in pressure cooker—fast release
Chickpeas	YES	40–60 minutes	18 minutes	22 minutes
Red kidney	YES	45–60 minutes	6 minutes	10 minutes
Borlotti beans	YES	45–60 minutes	7 minutes	12 minutes
Black beans	YES	40–50 minutes	3 minutes	5 minutes
Cannellini beans	YES	45–60 minutes	6 minutes	9 minutes
Lima/butter beans	YES	30–40 minutes	1–3 minutes	4 minutes
Adzuki beans	NO	30–40 minutes	2 minutes	4 minutes
Black-eyed peas	NO	30–45 minutes	3 minutes	5 minutes
Mung beans	NO	20–30 minutes	2 minutes	4 minutes
Split peas—yellow or green	NO	50–60 minutes	15–20 minutes	25–30 minutes
Lentils—brown, green, black	NO	15–20 minutes	6 minutes	8 minutes
Lentils—red split	NO	10–15 minutes	NO	NO

This table is a guide only that I have put together from many years of cooking legumes. Beans, chickpeas, and to a lesser degree lentils, vary greatly with cooking time depending on their age. It is best to buy small amounts from a shop with a high turnover and use them promptly to prevent the inconvenience of old dried beans that take 'forever' to cook.

If you find beans hard to digest because they cause an excess of wind, gas or bloating, first use smaller legumes like lentils, mung or adzuki beans, and start with a small amount, like ¼ of a cup when cooked. Cook them until they are very soft, and you could even try mashing them. Increase the amount consumed slowly (over several weeks) and as time goes by your body will adjust. When you feel you can digest the smaller beans and lentils easily, move up to the medium-sized ones like black beans, then finally try chickpeas and kidney beans.

soy

Although technically a legume, I have given soy its own category as not only is it a complete protein source, but it is one of the most widely studied food sources, both for environmental and health reasons.

Soy requires one tenth of the land to produce the same amount of protein from cattle. One cup of soybeans provides almost 50 percent of daily protein needs, along with almost 50 percent fibre, 50 percent of iron (or almost 100 percent for men) and 20 percent of calcium requirements.

Soybeans contain phytonutrients with antioxidant properties which help the soybean plant to thrive and confer health benefits to humans. The principal phytonutrients in soy are the isoflavones genistein and daidzein. They are 'phytoestrogens' or plant-estrogens with weak estrogen or anti-estrogen activity that can reduce the risk of estrogen-related cancers, like breast cancer. Isoflavones are powerful antioxidants and very effective tumour inhibitors. Soy also contains phytosterols (plant sterols), which compete with cholesterol for digestive absorption, reducing blood cholesterol levels. Regular soy intake is associated with reduced cardiovascular disease, partly due to lower LDL cholesterol levels and partly because the isoflavones have been shown to decrease arterial stiffness. Regular intake is also linked to improved bone health, reduced menopausal symptoms and reduced risk of prostate cancer.

Asian populations that consume soy regularly have a reduced incidence of breast cancer and menopausal symptoms compared with Western nations. Consumption during childhood and adolescence appears to have the biggest impact in reducing breast cancer risk.

Also note that Asian populations consume soy in whole or minimally processed forms such as tofu. They do not consume highly processed, isolated forms of soy that can be found in protein powders, bars and soy-meal alternatives available such as soy 'burgers' or 'sausages' in Western nations.

While we do not grow genetically modified (GM) soybeans in Australia, we do import some which are mostly used as animal feed. However, choosing organic soy products or checking for 'non-GM soy' listed on food labels can help you avoid GM soy. While there is no evidence currently to prove GM is unsafe, there understandably is some concern over potential human and environmental health risks from consuming and cultivating GM foods.

My preference for consuming soy is from whole or minimally processed foods such as edamame, other whole soybeans (often used in soy and linseed bread), soymilk (I choose an organic one), tofu and tempeh. Soy should be part of your vast variety of protein-rich foods, rather than the main or only source you eat.

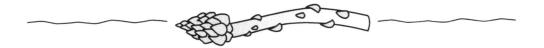

A note on 'mock meats'

Many meat alternatives contain highly processed ingredients and may also be very high in salt. Check the ingredients lists, look for whole food names you recognise and review the nutrition information panel for salt content before purchasing. Choose products with <120 mg of sodium per 100 grams.

Personally, I prefer to choose mostly whole plant proteins in their natural form—lentils, beans, chickpeas, soybeans, nuts and seeds—and have many quick, easy ways to make them into a meal.

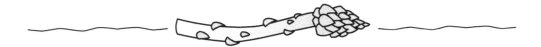

Nutrition and types of soy products

Soy food	Serving size	Protein (g)	Fat (g)	Sat fat (g)	Description	Culinary suggestions
Soy milk (calcium added)	1 cup (250 ml)	8–10	7	1	Milk alternative produced by soaking dried soy beans, mashing, then straining them. Most are fortified so contain the same amount of calcium as dairy milk which is 120 mg/100 ml. Check nutrition information panel to make sure	Use in place of dairy milk (straight swap) Has a lovely nutty flavour so goes well in coffee Also use with cereal, in smoothies and milkshakes and in cooking/baking
Edamame	½ cup (73 g)	17	9	1	Young green soy beans Available (usually frozen) in pods or podded	Eat as a snack (boil from frozen for 4–5 minutes first)—add to stir fries, salads, pasta or rice dishes or puree and make hummus or other dips/spreads
Soy beans	½ cup cooked (95 g)	14	8	1	Dried soy beans that you need to soak, then cook. May also be found pre-cooked in cans	Soups, salads, stir fries, casseroles, stews, curries, chilli, bread (soy and linseed bread)
Tofu —firm	½ cup (125 g)	15	9	1	Made by adding a coagulant to soy milk (similar to cheese making process) to get 'curds' and whey and is then pressed. The more well pressed the more whey is extracted, the firmer the tofu and the higher the protein and fat content	Bland taste so needs marinades, sauces or to be cooked in a dish like curries or casseroles where it can soak up flavour Use in stir fries or slice, marinade and pan-fry or bake to use in salads, sandwiches and burgers
Tofu —soft, silken	½ cup (125 g)	10	3	0	As above, but not pressed very much, has a higher liquid content and is much softer. Silken tofu has a lovely smooth texture and is my favourite form to use	Use to make dips, mayonaise and other creamy dressings Good egg replacement in quiches, fritattas or scrambled 'eggs' Makes great desserts like chocolate mousse
Tempeh	125 g	15	9	2	Whole soy beans combined with a grain and fermented into a firm 'cake'	Marinade and pan-fry, grill, barbecue or bake Use in stir fries and salads

NUTRITION DATA FROM FOODWORKS VERSION 8

NUTS AND SEEDS

Nuts and seeds are high in protein and contain important phytonutrients including flavonoids, phenolic acids, lignans, phytic acids and tocotrienols (part of vitamin E), which through their antioxidant effects can reduce your risk of cancer and cardiovascular disease.

NUTS' HEALTH BENEFITS

All nuts are a fabulous source of protein, fibre, healthy fats, vitamins, minerals and phytonutrients with antioxidant and anti-inflammatory properties.

Research has shown that this unique combination of healthy nutrients in nuts can reduce heart disease risk, lower cholesterol and help with weight management.

In particular, nuts are a great source of folate, niacin (vitamin B3), vitamin B6 (especially pistachios) and vitamin E (in particular almonds), magnesium, copper, zinc (cashews), selenium (Brazil nuts), phosphorus and potassium.

NUTS ARE INCREDIBLY VERSATILE

Add them to your breakfast bowl, muesli or granola, smoothies, salads, stir-fries, veggie burger mixes, pesto, dips and curry pastes, stuffing mixes, use in slices, cakes and biscuits either whole, roughly chopped or by grinding them into 'flour' first, puree into 'butter' and spread on sandwiches or toast for a quick breakfast or spread nut butter on crackers or fruit (apples, bananas) or veggies (celery, carrot) for a healthy snack.

You can of course eat nuts just as they are!

If you live in a warm, humid environment like most parts of Australia, it is best to store your nuts (and seeds) in the fridge. Once ground, store in the freezer. They can be used directly from the fridge or freezer.

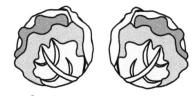

Did you know?

Peanuts are technically a legume whereas all other nuts are classified as tree nuts.

Walnuts are the only nuts that contain significant amounts of omega-3 fats, which are important for cognitive function (you may have noticed how walnuts resemble a brain), as well as reducing your risk of diabetes and heart disease. Walnuts are also particularly high in ellagic acid, a powerful antioxidant with anti-cancer potential, 98 percent of which is in the skin. Note that if your walnuts taste bitter, they are most likely rancid.

Pecans also contain omega-3 fats, but have much less than walnuts; roughly 10 percent that of walnuts.

Almonds are an excellent source of calcium for bone, teeth and general health as well as vitamin E, an antioxidant that supports the health of your blood, brain, eyes and skin.

Brazil nuts are a good source of selenium, a powerful antioxidant which may reduce your risk of cancer. Selenium is best sourced from food. An excess intake could occur from supplementation and can increase your cancer risk.

SEEDS' HEALTH BENEFITS

Although grains, legumes and nuts are all technically seeds, they are separated into their own culinary categories. So, I am referring to sunflower, pumpkin and sesame seeds along with chia, hemp seeds and linseeds.

Seeds contain everything needed to produce a plant. They are jam-packed with nutrients designed to help the seed sprout and grow.

Seeds are just as nutrient-rich as nuts, containing protein, carbohydrate, fat, fibre, vitamins, minerals and phytonutrients. Seeds also contain phytosterols, cholesterol-like compounds that can help lower LDL cholesterol levels.

Linseeds have the highest content of omega-3 fatty acids (ALA—alpha linolenic acid) of all the seeds, important for brain, nervous system and heart health. Linseeds contain lignans, a special type of soluble fibre that can reduce LDL cholesterol levels. They are also one of the richest sources of boron, a trace mineral important in bone health and are an excellent source of potassium and magnesium which can assist in lowering blood pressure. It is suggested that the body's ability to absorb of all of these wonderful nutrients is easier when the seeds are ground.

Chia seeds are also an excellent source of the omega-3 fatty acid ALA, followed closely by hemp seeds.

Hemp seeds have more protein than linseeds or chia seeds (2 tablespoons contain 7g). Hemp also contains gamma-linolenic acid and stearidonic acid, both essential fatty acids linked with reducing inflammation and pain in arthritis and lowering blood pressure.

Sunflower seeds are high in vitamin E, a powerful and important antioxidant and a good source of vitamin B6 important for healthy brain, immune and nervous system function.

> Seeds can be used in food in exactly the same way as nuts.

Tahini (sesame seed spread) can be used like peanut butter. Not only is it an important ingredient in hommus and baba ganoush, but simply mixed with a little lemon juice and garlic it makes a great dressing for salads and is delicious drizzled over roasted vegetables, in particular roasted pumpkin or roasted eggplant.

Sunflower seeds are a cost-effective way to make vegan 'milk', 'cream' and 'cheese' in place of nuts like almonds and cashews, which are often two to three times the price.

Seeds are best stored in the fridge when whole or freezer when ground. Ground linseeds can otherwise oxidise very quickly, so I prefer to buy them whole, grind myself and store in the freezer.

Plant Powered Protein Foods Nutrition composition per serving

Plant protein	Serving size	Carbs (g)	Protein (g)	Fat (g)	Sat fat (g)	Fibre (g)	Other relevant nutrients
Almonds	A handful, 30 g (approx. 23 nuts)	1	6	16	1	3	Calcium, Riboflavin, Niacin, Vitamin E, Plant sterols
Adzuki beans, cooked	½ cup (115 g)	28	9	0	0	8	Potassium, Magnesium, Folate, Vitamin B6
Black beans, cooked	½ cup (85 g)	19	8	0	0	6	Magnesium, Folate
Black eyed peas, cooked	½ cup (85 g)	19	7	0	0	5	Folate, Magnesium
Borlotti beans, cooked	½ cup (85 g)	19	7	0	0	5	Magnesium, Folate+
Brazil nuts	30 g (approx. 6–8 nuts)	1	4	20	4	3	Selenium, Magnesium, Phosphorus, Copper
Cannellini beans, cooked	½ cup (128 g)	16	8	1	0	8	Calcium, Potassium, Phosphorus
Cashews	A handful, 30 g (approx. 20 nuts)	5	5	15	3	2	Iron, Zinc, Niacin
Chia seeds	30 g (2 tbsp)	1	6	9	1	11	Omega–3 fatty acids (ALA)
Chickpeas, cooked	½ cup (100 g)	13	6	2	0	6	Potassium, Magnesium, Vitamin B6
Edamame, cooked	½ cup (73 g)	14	17	9	1	5	Omega–3 fatty acid (ALA) Calcium
Fava beans, cooked	½ cup (95 g)	13	7	<1	0	6	Potassium Copper

Plant protein	Serving size	Carbs (g)	Protein (g)	Fat (g)	Sat fat (g)	Fibre (g)	Other relevant nutrients
Hazelnuts	A handful, 30 g (approx. 21 nuts)	2	4	18	1	3	Folate Vitamin E
Hemp seeds	30 g (2½ tbsp)	0	9	17	2	2	Omega-3 fatty acid (ALA) Iron Magnesium Zinc
Kidney beans, cooked	½ cup (95 g)	14	7	1	0	7	Calcium Potassium Magnesium Vitamin B6
Lentils, cooked	½ cup (93 g)	9	7	0	0	4	Phosphorus Folate
Lima or Butter beans	½ cup (100 g)	10	6	0	0	5	Potassium Vitamin B6 Magnesium
Linseeds	30 g (2½ tablespoons)	9	5	13	1	8	Omega-3 fatty acid (ALA) Selenium
Macadamia nuts	30 g (approx. 10 nuts)	1	2	23	3	2	Thiamine Manganese
Mung beans, cooked	½ cup (85 g)	16	6	0	0	6	Potassium Magnesium Folate Vitamin B6
Peanuts	A handful, 30 g (approx. 40 'nuts')	3	7	14	2	2	Vitamin E Niacin Folate Magnesium Phosphorus
Peanut butter	30 g (1½ tbsp)	4	7	15	3	2	Vitamin E Niacin Folate Magnesium Phosphorus
Pecans	30 g (approx. 10–16 halves)	1	3	22	1	3	Manganese Polyphenols

Plant protein	Serving size	Carbs (g)	Protein (g)	Fat (g)	Sat fat (g)	Fibre (g)	Other relevant nutrients
Pine nuts	30 g (3 tbsp)	1	4	21	1	2	Zinc Phosphorus Niacin Vitamin E Manganese Plant sterols
Pistachios	A handful, 30 g (approx. 30+ nuts)	2	6	15	2	3	Potassium Vitamin B6 Copper Plant sterols Polyphenols
Pumpkin seeds	2 tbsp (30 g)	3	9	15	3	2	Zinc Potassium
Split peas, cooked	½ cup (98 g)	7	6	0	0	4	Thiamine
Soy beans, cooked	½ cup (100 g)	1	14	8	1	7	Potassium Magnesium Vitamin B6 Vitamin K
Sunflower seeds	30 g (2 tbsp)	1	8	15	1	3	Vitamin B6 Vitamin E
Tahini, sesame seed spread	30 g (1½ tbsp)	0	6	18	2	4	Calcium Iron Magnesium
Walnuts	1 handful, 30 g (approx. 15–20 halves)	1	4	21	1	2	Omega-3 fatty acid (ALA) Copper Polyphenols

DATA FROM FOODWORKS VERSION 8,
USDA FOOD COMPOSITION DATABASE AND
MANUFACTURERS' INFORMATION.

Note: Baked beans and tins of 4 or 5-bean mix are excellent protein sources for vegans.

You can also increase your protein intake by consuming flours made from legumes such as chickpea flour (also called besan) and lentil flour. These are commonly available in Australian supermarkets.

CARBOHYDRATES

Carbohydrates are the most misunderstood macronutrient, chiefly because they have been shunned by many popular 'fad' diets. Allow me to set the record straight on carbs.

The main thing you need to know is that carbohydrate foods provide your body with energy. In fact, carbohydrate is the preferred fuel source for all of the cells in your body, especially those in your brain. Carbohydrate foods mainly break down to glucose ('sugar') during digestion. Glucose is used as fuel by every cell in your body. Many carbohydrate-rich foods also contain important vitamins, minerals, fibre and antioxidants necessary for optimal health.

However not all carbohydrate foods are the same. Some are incredibly healthy, like lentils, whereas others, like lollipops, are not. Yet most people tend to lump all carbs in the same category.

Carbohydrate foods are broken down during digestion at different rates. Foods that are digested slowly to glucose are called low Glycemic Index (GI) foods and these slowly raise your blood sugar levels after eating. This is a good thing because most of us are not ultra-marathon runners so only use energy at a fairly slow rate. Lentils are a good example of a low GI food.

When blood sugar levels rise, your body produces a hormone called insulin which sweeps the sugar into the cells of your body where it is either used for energy or stored as glycogen in your muscle cells and the liver for later use.

If sugar levels rise slowly, the body is able to determine the amount of insulin needed and produce just enough to manage your sugar levels.

High GI foods like lollipops, on the other hand, are digested to sugar quickly. High sugar levels are dangerous to the body so large amounts of insulin are produced to help your body drop sugar levels just as quickly. This quick rise followed by a fast drop in sugar can affect your energy levels, mood and focus, and drives hunger.

High insulin levels in the blood encourage the conversion of sugar into fat for storage, which in turn can lead to weight gain. Eating this way often sets the scene for insulin resistance and increases the risk of developing type 2 diabetes. High insulin levels can also increase the risk of inflammation and certain hormone-related cancers.

High GI foods include highly-processed and refined foods such as white bread, most biscuits, cakes, sugary cereals, rice crackers and lollies. Sugary drinks are also high GI. Some less refined or unprocessed, natural foods are also high GI such as short grain white rice (jasmine rice), quick oats, watermelon and most potatoes. If eating these foods, combine with a low GI food, such as legumes, to slow digestion.

Many plant foods contain carbohydrate. These are legumes, wholegrains, all fruit and starchy vegetables—potato, sweet potato, corn, taro and yams. A few other vegetables contain smaller amounts of carbohydrate—pumpkin, fresh garden peas, parsnip, beetroot and swede—but rarely affect sugar levels unless eaten in large quantities. Salad greens, Asian stir-fry greens, green and other coloured vegetables are virtually carbohydrate free. Nuts and seeds also contain relatively little carbohydrate.

Most whole plant foods with carbohydrate are high in soluble fibre, which slows digestion, so are low GI. These foods therefore provide the perfect fuel for your body and brain. As well as beans, lentils, split peas, chickpeas, corn, sweet potato, whole rolled oats, barley and most fruit, choose low GI minimally processed foods, such as wholegrain or sourdough bread, pasta and muesli.

KETOSIS

When there is insufficient carbohydrate to fuel the brain, a condition called ketosis may result. Without carbohydrate, the body breaks down fat and by-products called ketone bodies build up in the blood. The brain, preferring glucose as its fuel, does not do well under these circumstances.

Ketosis can cause dizziness, headaches, nausea, fatigue, sleep problems and halitosis (bad breath). If it continues, dehydration, gout, hypotension (low blood pressure), electrolyte imbalance, and kidney and liver damage can occur.

Luckily the chance of ketosis occurring on a vegan intake is very limited. Carbohydrate Foods, their nutrition, composition and Glycemic Index (GI)

Plant carbohydrate	Serving size	Carbs (g)	Protein (g)	Fat (g)	Sat fat (g)	Fibre (g)	GI	LOW, MEDIUM OR HIGH GI
Amaranth, cooked	½ cup (123 g)	23	5	2	0	3	N/A	N/A
Barley, pearl, cooked	½ cup (79 g)	14	2	1	0	3	22	LOW
Bread—BurgenTM wholegrain	2 slices (84 g)	19	11	5	1	9	52	LOW
Bread—sourdough rye (e.g. Bill's Organic)	2 slices (40 g)	36	7	2	0	5	48	LOW
Buckwheat, cooked	½ cup (84 g)	17	3	1	0	2	54	LOW
Corn kernels	½ cup (87 g)	3	17	1	0	3	48	LOW
Millet, boiled	½ cup (87 g)	20	3	1	0	1	71	HIGH
Oats, whole rolled, raw	½ cup (40 g)	23	5	4	1	4	50	LOW
Polenta, cooked	½ cup (127 g)	11	1	0	0	1	68	MEDIUM
Potatoes—with skin, cooked	½ cup (83 g)	11	2	0	0	2	72–101	HIGH
Potatoes, Nicola (low GI varieties)	½ cup (120 g)	11	2	0	0	2	58	MEDIUM
Quinoa, cooked	½ cup (93 g)	20	4	2	0	3	51	LOW
Rice—brown, medium grain cooked	½ cup (90 g)	29	3	1	0	1	59	MEDIUM
Rice—white, long grain cooked	½ cup (95 g)	27	2	0	0	0	59	MEDIUM
Sweet potato—orange, cooked	½ cup (105 g)	15	2	2	44	2	61	MEDIUM
Sweet potato—purple, cooked	½ cup (105 g)	18	2	0	0	2	75	HIGH

DATA FROM FOODWORKS VERSION 8 AND GLYCEMIC INDEX www.GLYCEMICINDEX.COM

FIBRE

One of the most significant features of a plant-based intake is its high fibre content. In fact, fibre is only found in plant foods. To be healthy you need to eat more than 30 grams of fibre every day, which means consuming a reasonable quantity of plant foods. The average Australian consumes much less than the recommended levels, so their intake of fibre is inadequate.

Fibre keeps the digestive system healthy and prevents constipation. A high-fibre intake can also assist with weight management and appetite control, lower your risk of diabetes, heart disease and certain cancers (including bowel and breast), reduce inflammation, regulate immune function, reduce reflux and relieve some forms of irritable bowel syndrome (IBS).

WHAT IS FIBRE?

Fibre is the indigestible part of edible plant foods—fruit, vegetables, nuts, seeds, legumes and wholegrains—that your body cannot digest or absorb. Unlike other food components, such as fats, proteins or carbohydrates, which your body is able to break down and absorb, fibre is mostly resistant to these processes. Instead, it passes relatively unchanged through your stomach and small intestine. It then undergoes complete or partial fermentation in the large intestine (bowel or colon) and the remaining portion is then eliminated out of your body in the form of faeces (poo or 'number twos').

There are three different types of fibre. The most well-known are soluble and insoluble fibres. Resistant starch is the third and most-recently recognised type of fibre. You need to consume a balance of all three to receive the beneficial effects that each offers.

Soluble fibre dissolves in water to form a gel-like matter which helps to soften the faeces, helping it pass through the gut more easily, thereby keeping you 'regular'. It slows the digestion and absorption of carbohydrate foods, which helps to keep blood sugar levels steady and can lower LDL cholesterol levels. All fruit and vegetables contain soluble fibre. Legumes in particular are an excellent source of soluble fibre, along with oats, barley, psyllium husks and seeds, especially chia and linseeds.

Insoluble fibre adds bulk to faeces and stimulates peristalsis (contraction and relaxation) in the intestines to keep things moving, pushing matter through for elimination. This helps to prevent constipation and associated problems such as diverticulitis and haemorrhoids. Insoluble fibre is found in the skin of all fruit and vegetables. It is the main fibre in wheat and is also found in most other grains and legumes.

Resistant starch is the part of starchy food that resists normal digestion in the stomach and small intestine, arriving unchanged in the large intestine (bowel). It has been extensively studied by the CSIRO for its ability to vastly reduce bowel cancer risk.

Bacteria that inhabit the large bowel (part of our 'gut microbiome') break down (ferment) and change resistant starch into short-chain fatty acids (SCFAs), in particular butyrate, which nourishes the lining of the cell wall and helps protect against bowel cancer. SCFAs play a role in lowering blood cholesterol levels, improving insulin sensitivity and blood glucose control. They also help improve immunity and maintain the pH of the large intestine at a level supportive for growth of healthy bacteria. You will find resistant starch in legumes, barley, oats, corn, green bananas as well as cooked and cooled potato, pasta and rice.

Fibre type	Good food sources	How to increase your intake
Soluble	Oats Psyllium Seeds Legumes—lentils, split peas, beans, chickpeas Barley Vegetable and fruit flesh	Include oats in breakfast as porridge or muesli Add psyllium, linseeds or chia seeds to your breakfast cereal or smoothie Add legumes to soups, salads and casseroles Make salad out of cooked barley or add to soups Include vegetables and fruit in meals and snacks
Insoluble	Wholegrain bread Wholegrain cereal Wheat and rice bran Wholegrains Nuts Vegetable and fruit skin	Choose wholegrain bread Choose wholegrain cereals over more refined choices Add rice bran to cakes and muffin mixes Use brown rice in place of white Include nuts as a healthy snack Eat the skin on fruit and veggies (where possible)
Resistant Starch	Legumes especially chickpeas Barley Corn Banana (lightly ripe) Cooked and cooled pasta, rice and potato	Spread hommus on crackers for a healthy snack Add chickpeas to salads, soups and casseroles Eat fresh corn on the cob when in season Have a banana as a snack Make a salad out of cooled potatoes

FIBRE AND THE GUT MICROBIOME

Your gut is home to trillions of bacteria and this is a very good thing! This diverse microbe community lives happily with you in a mutually beneficial relationship where they rely on you for food and shelter and you need them for functions critical to your health and wellbeing.

The term 'microbiota' refers to the collection of micro-organisms that live in your gut, mainly comprised of bacteria, Along with their DNA, these micro-organisms form your microbiome or 'gut flora'. They reside mostly in the large intestine and play a key role in digestion and help with the absorption and synthesis of nutrients. They also influence your metabolism, body weight, immune regulation, brain function and mood. Your microbiome is unique to you, like a bacterial fingerprint, and research suggests that a diverse range of gut bacteria is very important for optimal health.

Your gut microbiome begins to develop in very early life and is influenced by birth delivery method, genetics, age, stress, exposure to infection or illness, environment, medication use and diet. In fact, what you eat can quickly change the type of bacteria in your gut.

DYSBIOSIS

Intestinal dysbiosis is an imbalance in your microbial ecosystem, where pathogenic (bad) bacteria begin to dominate over non-pathogenic or beneficial bacteria. Such changes in gut flora are associated with the development of irritable bowel syndrome (IBS). Dysbiosis can also compromise intestinal permeability, cause a 'leaky gut' and increase susceptibility to inflammatory conditions such as inflammatory bowel diseases (IBD) or bowel cancer, asthma, metabolic syndrome, cardiovascular disease and obesity.

PROBIOTICS

A probiotic is a specific strain of bacteria or yeast that promotes health for the host and competes with, thus protects against, disease-causing bacteria. Most of the 'friendly' bacteria that make up your intestinal flora are probiotics. They are also found in some fermented foods like yoghurt, sauerkraut (unpasteurised), miso and kimchi.

PREBIOTICS

Prebiotics are fibre-rich foods that pass through the upper part of your gut undigested and end up as a food source for your beneficial microbes (probiotics), keeping them happy and supporting diversity. Most whole plant foods that contain soluble fibre and all foods with resistant starch are prebiotics. Prebiotic foods include legumes—lentils, dried beans, split peas, soy beans and chickpeas, globe and Jerusalem artichokes, chicory root, bananas, endives, garlic, leeks, onions, parsnips, savoy cabbage, almonds, linseeds, unrefined wheat, rye, oats, barley, polenta and corn.

Eating a high-fibre intake that includes plenty of colourful plant foods will ensure a richer and more diverse gut microbiome, keeping it and you healthy, balanced and functioning optimally.

ANTIOXIDANTS

Antioxidants are substances that protect the cells in your body from damage caused by oxidation (exposure to oxygen). Phytonutrients are naturally occurring compounds in all plant foods, closely associated with the fibre components, that amongst their many benefits can function as antioxidants and help protect against many health problems.

Antioxidants can protect you from ageing, inflammation, oxidative stress and many chronic illnesses. They prevent cellular damage by removing 'free radicals', controlling free radical production and inhibiting other negative oxidation reactions that occur as a part of normal metabolism.

Free radicals are a by-product of normal body cell functions and can also come from outside sources, such as pollution, pesticides, drugs, fumes, lead, mercury and radiation, as well as lifestyle factors such as smoking, stress, alcohol, excess sunlight and poor food choices. They don't actually like being 'free' and prefer to latch on to other substances; however, when they do so they can cause damage. When free-radical damage goes unchecked by antioxidants, it can cause significant harm to cells which can lead to disease.

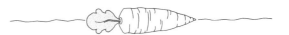

Antioxidants are found in all plant-based foods such as fruit, vegetables, legumes, nuts, seeds and wholegrains. They are also abundant in herbs and spices. Many vitamins, for example, vitamins C, E and beta-carotene (the precursor to vitamin A) as well as minerals such as selenium, zinc and copper are antioxidants.

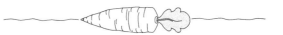

INFLAMMATION

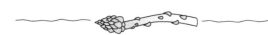

Research has linked chronic systemic inflammation to almost every major disease. Inflammation is present in auto-immune conditions, such as joint inflammation and arthritis, and is implicated in asthma and allergies, cardiovascular disease and diabetes. It accelerates the ageing process, encourages weight gain and can make weight loss more difficult.

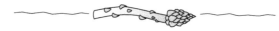

Most of us have experienced inflammation in the form of a bite, pimple or rash. It is a natural body reaction to infection and injury. Immune response signals increase blood flow to get more immune cells and nutrients to the affected site to fight infection and repair the body's cells and tissues. You would notice this as pain, swelling, heat and redness. This type of acute inflammation is a normal and necessary part of the body's defence mechanisms and healing process. It helps protect you against life-threatening situations by eliminating bacteria, viruses, and altered self-cells that could otherwise lead to disease. Sometimes inflammation doesn't end when it is supposed to. Instead, it sticks around in a low-grade, chronic form, silently targeting healthy tissues, causing damage and disease. Inflammation is fuelled by many factors, including stress, lack of sleep, high blood pressure or sugar levels, abdominal obesity, cigarette smoke and, to a large degree, what you eat.

The good news is that a plant-based intake has an anti-inflammatory effect in the human body.

Whole plant foods contain powerful antioxidants that interact with, and downregulate, genes that promote inflammation. In fact, a plant-based intake is very effective at preventing inflammation and can also help dampen any active inflammation.

PHYTONUTRIENTS

The word 'phytonutrient' comes from the Greek 'phyto' meaning 'plant', and 'nutrient' meaning 'vital substances for health'. Plants typically produce several phytonutrients as they act as a protective mechanism against environmental stressors; the more environmental stressors, the more phytonutrients a plant produces.

Phytonutrients are non-essential nutrients, meaning that they are not required by the human body for sustaining life, but they are necessary for optimal health as they provide health benefits way beyond those that essential nutrients can provide. It is these natural compounds that give plants their distinctive colour, flavour and smell. Thousands of different phytonutrients, each with unique disease-preventing properties, have been identified. Most likely, there are many more still to be discovered.

Phytonutrients are powerful health-promoting substances to include in your intake. There is growing evidence that they play a crucial role in helping to maintain human health and prevent a number of diseases, such as cardiovascular disease, diabetes, neurodegenerative conditions like Alzheimer's, as well as macular degeneration and many cancers.

The reported health benefits from phytonutrients are only available when eating plant foods, not when supplements are used. Phytonutrients appear to work synergistically with the vitamins, minerals, fibre and other important nutrients found in plants. The crucial interaction of hundreds of different nutrients when eating a combination of food appears to be lost when taken in pill form. Not surprisingly, a pill cannot do what eating real, whole food can!

Fruit and vegetables tend to be categorised into five colour groups, according to the phytonutrients they contain. Each colour provides various health benefits and no one colour is superior to another. Typically, the deeper the colour, the more phytonutrients present in the food. Notable exceptions are cauliflower, garlic and onions, which contain plenty of these incredibly healthy substances.

Note also that the colour of a food does not necessarily mean it contains only one type of phytonutrient. Most plant foods contain multiple phytonutrients.

Research suggests that diversity is more important than amount if you want to gain the most benefit from your phytonutrient intake. Different phytonutrients have unique health benefits thanks to their specific chemical structures, but they work best as a team to protect your health. In other words, you need to include fruit and vegetables from each of the colour groups every day ('eat the rainbow'), to meet your body's needs for all of the different phytonutrients. Good news considering it would be pretty boring if you just ate carrots or broccoli every day!

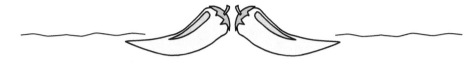

To maximise your daily intake of phytonutrients:

❖ Eat phytonutrient-rich foods frequently throughout the day. This helps keep blood levels of these components constant and ultimately more effective

❖ Eat at least five to seven servings a day of vegetables

❖ Eat at least two servings of fruit

❖ Create your meal around vegetables. Fill at least half your plate with different colours

❖ Include the fruit and vegetable skins (those that are edible of course) and choose organic where possible. The skins are a concentrated source of phytonutrients.

❖ Regularly include a wide range of wholegrains and legumes in your intake as they also contain important phytonutrients

It's okay to cook your vegetables because most phytonutrients are heat-stable. In fact, cooking can increase bio-availability of some phytonutrients, for example, lycopene in tomatoes.

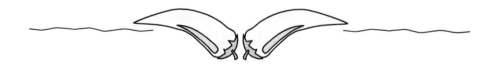

Phytonutrient Guide

Colour	Phytonutrient	Health Benefits	Foods
Red	Lycopene	Helps control high blood pressure. Reduces risk of heart attacks and cancer, especially prostate	Fresh tomatoes and tomato-based products—bioavailability increases when tomatoes are cooked
	Anthocyanins	Reduces risk of cancer, diabetes, heart disease and Alzheimer's	Strawberries, raspberries, red apples, red cabbage
Yellow And Orange	Beta-carotene (dark orange)	Convers to vitamin A in body, integral for vision, immune function and healthy skin. Reduces risk of heart disease and cancer	Carrots, pumpkin, sweet potatoes, mangoes, apricots, peaches
	Bioflavanoids (yellow-orange)	Help maintain good vision, teeth/bones and healthy skin	Oranges, grapefruits, lemons, pears
Green	Lutein (yellow-green and leafy greens)	Helps maintain good vision. Reduces risk of cataracts and age-related macular degeneration	Kale, spinach, leafy greens, lettuce, peas, kiwifruit
	Indoles (cruciferous vegetables)	Reduces risk of cancers including breast, prostate and bowel cancer	Broccoli, cabbage, cauliflower, kale, watercress, Brussels sprouts
White And Brown	Allicin	Helps lower high blood pressure and LDL cholesterol Reduces risk of heart attacks and cancer. Also anti-bacterial and anti-viral properties	Garlic, onions, leeks, spring onions, chives
Purple	Anthocyanins	Reduce risk of cancer, heart disease, diabetes and age-related memory loss	Blueberries, blackberries, blackcurrants, purple grapes Spanish (red) onion and red (purple) cabbage
	Phenolics	May slow effects of ageing	Eggplant, plums, prunes, raisins

ADAPTED FROM THE CANCER PROJECT (2010)

FAT

Most plant-based foods contain little or no fat and no plant food contains cholesterol. Most plant foods are low in saturated fat. Saturated fat is associated with: increasing cholesterol levels in the body and heart disease risk; increased risk of insulin resistance; type 2 diabetes and some cancers.

There are some plant foods that are higher in fat, but they contain mostly healthier mono- and polyunsaturated fats which are required by the body to stay healthy. These are nuts, seeds, avocado, olives and soybeans.

There are a few plant foods high in saturated fat. Coconut is one but consumed in its whole food form is relatively harmless. Cocoa butter, extracted from cacao beans, is high in saturated fat and may raise blood cholesterol levels. Palm oil or palm kernel oil not only is high in saturated fat, but most palm oil is not sustainably sourced, so best avoided.

Soy beans and tofu, walnuts, linseeds, chia seeds and, to a lesser extent, leafy green vegetables and some legumes, including red kidney beans and chickpeas, are all good sources of the essential omega-3 fatty acids which your body cannot produce, but are essential for a healthy heart, brain, joints, vision and even your mood. It is a good idea to include these foods daily.

Saturated fat	Monounsaturated fat	Polyunsaturated fat
Butter and full fat dairy Skin and fat in meat Coconut oil Palm oil Most processed foods	Extra virgin olive oil Macadamia oil Avocadoes Most nuts including peanuts and peanut butter Most seeds including tahini	Essential fatty acids (EFAs) Omega-3 and omega-6 Omega-6—essential; small amounts needed Best sourced from whole plant foods, such as nuts and seeds. Try to avoid concentrated sources like vegetable oils (sunflower, cottonseed) and polyunsaturated margarines
Best to limit as may increase cholesterol levels and risk of cardiovascular disease, diabetes and dementia	Present in canola margarine and olive oil margarine but these are not recommended as they are heavily processed	Omega-3—essential Fatty fish and most seafood Linseeds and flaxseed oil Chia seeds, Hemp seeds Walnuts Soy and soy products

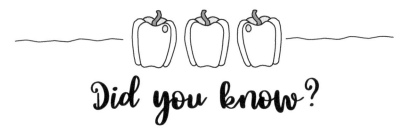

Did you know?

Olive oil is made from crushing and pressing the whole olive fruit—pits and all—as opposed to a seed (such as canola seeds, which is the source of canola oil) or the germ (corn). Olives are a fruit and they provide a large amount of plant antioxidants called 'polyphenols', which are scarce in other oils derived from seeds or vegetables.

Extra virgin olive oil, also known as 'cold pressed', (no heat was used during the pressing of the olives), is from the first press of the olives. It is the purest and least processed of all the olive oils, contains the most antioxidants (polyphenols) and is the most flavoursome. The high antioxidant content also helps protect the oil, keeping it stable when heated so extra virgin olive oil is the best oil with which to cook.

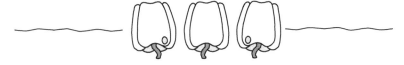

POLYUNSATURATED FATS

Polyunsaturated fats or fatty acids (PUFAs) are fats that your body cannot make, so it is essential that you obtain these from the foods you eat. They are necessary for proper brain and nervous system function, vision and healthy cell formation and growth. They also produce hormone-like substances called 'eicosanoids' that regulate certain body functions. While they are both essential, getting the right balance between omega-3 and omega-6 intake is most important.

Both omega-3 and omega-6 use the same conversion pathway in the body, so getting too much of one will reduce conversion of the other. Due to changes in food production and processing methods over the past 50 years, the average person's intake now provides a much higher level of omega 6 relative to omega 3 (estimated between 12:1 and 25:1), which may increase risk of heart disease, diabetes, certain cancers as well as immune and inflammatory conditions.

The optimal omega 6: omega 3 ratio is between 4:1 and 2:1

OMEGA-3 FATS

Omega-3 fats are vital for optimal health; they are incorporated into every cell, tissue and organ in your body from the heart and brain to the eyes, lungs, muscles, reproductive organs, blood vessels and joints and have strong anti-inflammatory effects. They can reduce inflammation and symptoms associated with arthritis, especially rheumatoid arthritis, eczema and auto-immune conditions like psoriasis. They help lower triglyceride levels, prevent your blood from clotting unnecessarily and can lower high blood pressure, thus reducing your risk of cardiovascular disease. Research shows that a higher intake of omega 3 fats is beneficial for those with heart disease or a strong family history of heart disease, high triglyceride levels, diabetes, inflammatory or autoimmune conditions.

There are four main omega-3 fats: DHA (docosahexaenoic acid), EPA (eicosapentaenoic acid), DPA (docosapentaenoic acid) and ALA (alpha-linolenic acid). DHA and EPA are the most extensively studied and well-understood omega-3 fats, found primarily in oily fish, but actually originate from marine plants, mostly microalgae. DPA, along with smaller amounts of EPA and DHA, is found in animal products, such as organic and some free-range eggs, organic chicken and beef, and wild fish.

The only truly 'essential' omega-3 fat is ALA, which is derived from plants. With sufficient intake, your body can convert ALA into DHA and EPA. The efficiency at which it does this is variable however, and is mainly determined by genetics, sex, age and dietary composition.

GUIDELINES FOR VEGANS

In Australia, adequate intakes suggested for ALA are 1.3 g/day for men and 0.8 g/day for women, and for long-chain n-3 PUFAs (EPA/DHA) are 160 mg/day for men and 90 mg/day for women. Whereas, to reduce your chronic disease risk, an average daily intake of 2 g of ALA and 610 mg/day for men and 430 mg/day for women of EPA/DHA is suggested.

Since intakes of DHA/EPA are virtually absent in vegans, it is suggested to double the current recommendations of ALA if no direct sources of EPA and DHA are consumed. In other words, aim for an average daily intake of 4 g of ALA. You can achieve this by eating more sources of ALA, such as walnuts, linseeds (best ground), chia seeds, hemp seeds, tofu, leafy green vegetables and beans. See table on the following page which lists amounts found in these foods.

To enhance your intake of omega-3, limit consumption of omega-6 fats in extracted/ concentrated forms like vegetable oils made from corn, sunflower, safflower, soy bean and grapeseed as well as polyunsaturated margarines. Check food labels for these oils. While you need some omega-6 fats, eating too much limits your body's ability to benefit from omega 3 fats.

Avoid foods that contain trans fats since they interfere with EPA and DHA production. Trans fats are found in deep-fried foods and foods containing 'partially hydrogenated' oils or vegetable fat.

Food	Serving size	ALA (grams)
Chia seeds	1 tablespoon, 14 g	2.5
Linseeds	1 tablespoon whole, 14 g 1 tablespoon ground*, 9 g	3.3 2.1
Hemp seeds	1 tablespoon, 12 g	1.0
Walnuts	¼ cup, 30 g	1.9
Tofu, firm	½ cup, 125 g	0.5
Edamame (green soy beans)	½ cup, 95 g	0.4
Soybean, mature, cooked	½ cup, 95 g	0.4
Red kidney, borlotti, black beans, black eyed peas, cooked	½ cup, approx. 95 g	0.2
Flaxseed (linseed) oil	1 teaspoon, 5 ml	2.5
Walnut oil	1 teaspoon, 5 ml	0.5

DATA FROM FOODWORKS VERSION 8, USDA FOOD COMPOSITION DATABASE, DIETITIANS OF CANADA FOOD SOURCES OF OMEGA 3 FAT FACTS SHEET AND MANUFACTURERS' INFORMATION.

*IT IS SUGGESTED THAT OMEGA-3 FATS ARE BETTER ABSORBED FROM GROUND LINSEEDS DUE TO THE HARD COATING ON WHOLE SEEDS.

Vegans with increased needs, for example, while pregnant and breastfeeding, or reduced conversion ability (elderly or those with chronic disease such as diabetes) would benefit from DHA and EPA supplements derived from microalgae.
A supplement of 200-300mg/day of DHA and EPA is recommended.

For more information and to find out what is right for you, ask your doctor or dietitian.

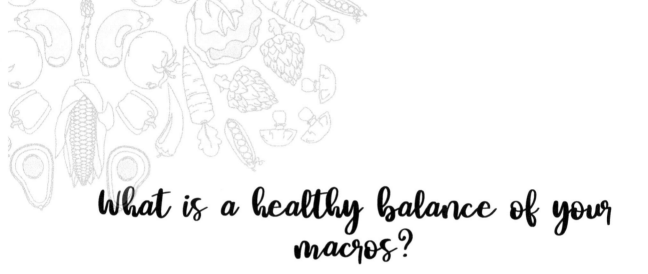

What is a healthy balance of your macros?

There is no hard and fast rule, but approximately:
15-25 percent protein
45-65 percent carbohydrate
20-35 percent fat

Notes

know where to find
your micronutrients

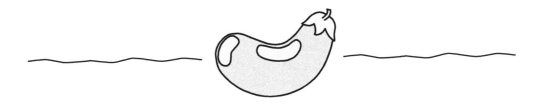

Vitamins and minerals are micronutrients—
essential elements required in small quantities
throughout your life. They orchestrate numerous
functions necessary for normal growth,
development, to maintain health (prevent disease)
and overall wellbeing.

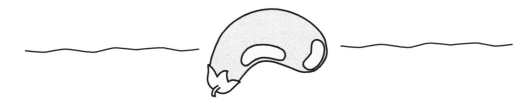

VITAMINS

Vitamins are vital for life. They are necessary for normal growth and functioning of the body and they help you metabolise macronutrients. Vitamins help regulate metabolism by acting as enzymes or co-enzymes that facilitate biochemical reactions in your body. Many vitamins are antioxidants or form an integral part of the structure of proteins, hormones and blood.

> Vitamins are essential, organic nutrients required in tiny amounts and perform specific functions in growth, reproduction and maintenance of health and life

There are two types of vitamins; fat-soluble and water-soluble. Fat-soluble vitamins include vitamins A, D, E and K. When you consume more than your body needs in any given day, the excess is stored in fatty tissue and the liver until needed. Therefore, fat-soluble vitamins can be eaten in large amounts once in a while and continue to meet your needs over time. All other vitamins are water-soluble. When digested and absorbed, they move directly into the blood and any excess is excreted in urine. This means you need to have a regular intake of these vitamins. The only exception is vitamin B12.

It is best to obtain your vitamins (other than B12) from food as they are in the most biologically available form, the correct amount and coincide with other complementary nutrients that have a synergistic health benefit. Vitamin supplementation cannot compete with a nutritious intake of whole fresh food. There is also little risk of overdosing on vitamins from food. Supplements however can provide excess quantities which can be harmful on their own or disturb the balance of other vitamins and minerals, for example, folate supplements can mask the symptoms of B12 deficiency.

Given that a well-planned vegan intake based on whole foods would typically include many more vitamin-rich foods such as fruit, vegetables, legumes, nuts and seeds than an omnivorous diet, you have virtually no risk of vitamin deficiencies, other than vitamin B12 which is only available in animal products or as a supplement. For that reason, I have separated vitamin B12 and discussed it in length here. I have put all other vitamins into two separate tables; one each for the water-soluble and fat-soluble vitamins.

VITAMIN B12

Plant foods provide all the nutrients necessary for optimal health, apart from vitamin B12.

Vitamin B12 is a very important nutrient. Vitamin B12 works together with folate (another B vitamin), depending on each other for activation. Together they keep nerve cells and blood cells healthy and are involved in the formation of the genetic material DNA and RNA. Vitamin B12 is also involved in the metabolism of carbohydrates and fats.

Vitamin B12 deficiency may counteract some benefits of eating healthy. If not detected early it can become serious, resulting in:

❖ Pernicious anaemia where the body produces abnormally-shaped red blood cells that can't carry oxygen, so can't function properly. Symptoms include tiredness and weakness. A smooth, painful, red tongue and/or mouth ulcers can also be a sign of pernicious anaemia

❖ Peripheral neuropathy, an irreversible nerve damage causing numbness, tingling or 'pins and needles' in your feet and hands that can progress to paralysis

❖ Increased levels of an artery-damaging compound called 'homocysteine', greatly increasing your risk of cardiovascular disease

❖ Other issues such as hypersensitive skin; muscle weakness; problems with balance and co-ordination; eyesight problems; depression; confusion; and memory loss (may even be misdiagnosed as Alzheimer's disease!).

Vitamin B12 is only found naturally in foods from animal sources—it is produced by their bacteria. Sources for vegans are therefore limited and a vitamin B12 supplement is usually needed. Check if any processed foods you use are fortified because vitamin B12 is added to some plant-based milks (often in soymilk but check labels) as well as many soy-based and other vegan products. These may be a reliable source. If 'fortified' or 'enriched', nutritional yeast can be a good source too. Note that some foods such as tempeh, miso, spirulina and seaweed contain B12, but it is an inactive, unavailable form that cannot be used by the body. Microwave heating inactivates vitamin B12.

To be sure you're getting your 2.4 mcg/day, you may consider taking a vitamin B12 supplement. You can take supplements either daily or weekly. Your body absorbs vitamin B12 more efficiently in frequent small amounts, so the less frequently you consume it, the more you will need. Note that vitamin B12 is not toxic at high amounts because your body removes what is not needed. Vitamin B12 supplements are not made from animal-based products so are suitable for vegans.

Adults require 2.4 mcg/day of vitamin B12. Slightly more is required when pregnant or breastfeeding.

WHAT AFFECTS B12 ABSORPTION?

Intrinsic factor (IF) is made by the parietal cells in the stomach and is necessary for vitamin B12 to be absorbed in the small intestine. In some people, IF is not produced in sufficient amounts, and even with adequate intake, they cannot absorb enough vitamin B12. Ability to absorb vitamin B12 may also decrease with age, if you have low stomach acid (due to taking medications like Nexium, Somac or Zantac) or if you are taking metformin (diabetes medication). Absorption can also be affected by certain autoimmune conditions like Crohn's disease or coeliac disease, and also may be reduced after gastric sleeve and other types of gastric (stomach) surgery.

If in doubt, it is best to get a blood test to check your vitamin B12 levels. I usually suggest prior to or soon after making changes to your intake (becoming vegan) to have a base-line blood test and follow-up tests (usually for iron as well) every 3 to 6 months within the first year to check that your intake and absorption of these nutrients is adequate. Although it may take up to three years to develop a deficiency as the body recycles much of its vitamin B12, over time you may see a decline in your levels.

NUTRITIONAL YEAST

Nutritional yeast, also called 'savoury yeast flakes' (comes powdered or in flakes) is a seasoning that has a nutty, umami flavour that can give a Parmesan-like kick to soups, sauces, pastas, salads, risottos, other rice, grain or legume dishes, bean stews, pesto, tofu scramble, nut roasts, stuffing and vegetable dishes.

Nutritional yeast is very different from the yeast used in bread. It is made from Saccharomyces cerevisiae or S. cerevisiae, a single-celled organism which is grown on molasses, then harvested, washed and dried with heat to "deactivate" it. Because it's inactive, it doesn't froth or grow like baker's yeast does so has no leavening ability. It is a member of the fungi family, like mushrooms.

Nutritional yeast, as the name implies, contains many valuable nutrients. It is a very good source of B vitamins (like thiamine, niacin, folate, B6) except for B12, however is often fortified or enriched with vitamin B12 (don't assume, always check). Nutritional yeast contains magnesium, copper and manganese, zinc and fibre. It is also a complete protein, however as it is usually eaten in such small amounts it cannot effectively contribute to your daily protein requirements.

It is a great seasoning alternative because it is low in sodium, and especially recommended if you're trying to cut down on your salt intake.

Research has shown that S. cerevisiae, the strain of yeast in nutritional yeast, can support the immune system and reduce inflammation resulting from bacterial infections.

To show you an example of what it contains, here is the nutritional breakdown of the nutritional yeast I use, purchased from Honest To Goodness. As you can see, 1 tablespoon (approx. 10 g) will supply 11 mcg of vitamin B12 which is one-tenth of the amount supplied by 100 grams.

Nutritional information	Average per 100 g	Average per serve 10 g
Energy	1640 kJ	164 kJ
Protein	47 g	4.7 g
Fat – total	4.8 g	0.5 g
Fat – saturated	0.9 g	0 g
Carbohydrate	19.8 g	2.0 g
Sugars	12.4 g	1.2 g
Sodium	315 mg	32 mg
Thiamine (B1)	14 mg	1.4 mg
Riboflavin (B2)	55 mg	5.5 mg
Niacin (B3)	266 mg	27.0 mg
Pantothenic acid (B5)	99 mg	10 mg
Pyridoxine (B6)	23 mg	2.3 mg
Biotin (B7)	23 mcg	2.3 mcg
Folic acid (B9)	2150 mcg	215 mcg
Cobalamin (B12)	108 mcg (fortified)	11 mcg (fortified)

NUTRITION INFORMATION SOURCED FROM NUTRITIONAL
YEAST FOOD PACKAGE BY HONEST TO GOODNESS.
FOR MORE INFORMATION VISIT
HTTPS://WWW.GOODNESS.COM.AU/NUTRITIONAL-YEAST-FLAKES-TOASTED-150G

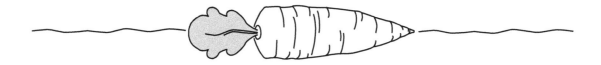

WATER-SOLUBLE VITAMINS

There are nine essential B vitamins that work together as a team (B group or B-complex vitamins). They depend on each other to function optimally. Together they convert food (carbohydrates, protein and fat) to energy that you use throughout the day; a process known as 'energy metabolism'. Some have numbers associated with them and some don't, which is just due to when they were discovered.

B vitamins other than B12 tend to be in the same foods—wholegrains (note, when grains are refined, most of the B vitamins along with important minerals and fibre are removed), legumes, nuts, seeds, vegetables and nutritional yeast.

The B-complex vitamins and vitamin C are water-soluble, which means they dissolve easily upon entering the body. Many are also sensitive to heat and can be lost in cooking water when boiled or blanched, so it's best to steam your veggies. Since the body cannot store them, ideally water-soluble vitamins should be consumed daily.

Deficiencies of vitamins can cause diseases such as beriberi (lack of vitamin B1) often due to heavy alcohol intake, pellagra (lack of vitamin B3) characterised by dermatitis, diarrhoea and mental disturbance (dementia), birth defects (folate) and scurvy (lack of vitamin C) which causes swollen and bleeding gums, and bruising.

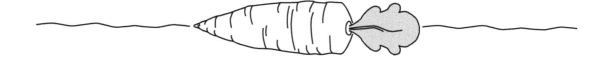

Vitamin	Needed for	Recommended daily intake (RDI)	Vegan food sources
B1 (thiamine) *easily destroyed by heat	Helps release energy from carbohydrates Needed for proper working of the heart, digestive and nervous systems (nerve cells) Important for growth and appetite	Women: 1.1 mg Men: 1.2 mg	Yeast extract (e.g. Vegemite™) Wheat germ and bran Wholegrain products Nuts Sesame seeds Legumes Peas
B2 (riboflavin) *stable to heat	Important for growth and repair of tissues Supports healthy skin and eyes Helps release energy from food (energy metabolism) Metabolism of carbohydrates, protein and fat	Women: <70: 1.1 mg >70: 1.3 mg Men <70: 1.3 mg >70: 1.6 mg	Yeast extract (e.g. Vegemite™) Nutritional yeast Almonds Peanuts Mushrooms Sweet Potato Wholegrain products Dark leafy green vegetables including broccoli, spinach, asparagus and peas
B3 (niacin) Can be made in the body from tryptophan *fairly heat resistant	Helps to release energy from food Essential for growth Suppresses inflammation Important for nervous system and digestive health Used to treat high LDL cholesterol and triglyceride levels	Women: 14 mg Men: 16 mg Upper limit is 35 mg	Nutritional yeast Peanuts Legumes Sunflower seeds Mushrooms Leafy green vegetables Avocado Peas Sweet potato Wholegrains

Vitamin	Needed for	Recommended daily intake (RDI)	Vegan food sources
B5 (Pantothenic acid) *fairly heat resistant	Helps release energy from carbohydrates and fat Involved in the formation of haemoglobin (the central part of red blood cells which carries oxygen), neurotransmitters and steroid hormones Intestinal bacteria may synthesise this vitamin, further contributing to your intake	Women: 4 mg Men: 6 mg	Yeast Yeast extract (e.g. Vegemite™) Soy beans Nuts Wholegrains including brown rice and barley Broccoli Mushrooms Avocado
B6 (pyridoxine) Stored in muscle tissue *easily destroyed by heat	Helps assist enzymes that metabolise amino acids Assists in making red blood cells Important for brain function, synthesis of key neurotransmitters, immune health and steroid hormone activity	Up to 50 years: 1.3 mg Women >50: 1.5 mg Men >50: 1.7 mg	Nutritional and brewer's yeast Soybeans and soy products Seeds Nuts Wholegrains including rice and barley Avocado Non-citrus fruit Seaweed
Folate (folic acid) *destroyed by high temperatures	Works together with vitamin B12 to build DNA and new cells, especially those lining the GI tract Formation of red blood cells Helps in amino acid metabolism Breaks down homocysteine and reduces cardiovascular disease risk Keeps the nervous system healthy Important in early pregnancy to prevent neural tube defects	400 mcg *requires adequate iron and vitamin C levels for absorption	Yeast extract (e.g. Vegemite™) Nutritional yeast Green leafy vegetables Avocado, Peas Asparagus, Okra Wholegrains Legumes Sunflower seeds Nuts (especially hazelnuts) Strawberries Oranges

Vitamin	Needed for	Recommended daily intake (RDI)	Vegan food sources
Biotin *fairly heat resistant	Energy metabolism Glycogen synthesis Helps process fat and protein Important for growth and nerve cell function	Women: 2.5 mcg Men: 30 mcg	Oats Wholegrains Legumes Soybeans Mushrooms Nuts and Seeds Biotin is also made by bacteria in the intestine
Choline *fairly heat resistant	Component of cell membranes and the neurotransmitter acetylcholine Important in fat and bile metabolism Your body can make choline from the amino acid methionine	Women:425 mg Men: 550 mg	Lecithin Wheat germ Brewer's yeast Legumes, especially soy beans and peanuts Wholegrains Nuts Leafy green vegetables
B12 (cyanocobalamin) *fairly heat resistant except in microwaves	Works together with folate Proper formation of red blood cells Formation of nerve cells and DNA Metabolism of carbohydrates and fat	2.4 mcg	Fortified foods Note that many foods contain an inactive form Supplements are usually required

Vitamin	Needed for	Recommended daily intake (RDI)	Vegan food sources
Vitamin C (ascorbic acid) *vulnerable to heat	Powerful antioxidant which defends the body against free radical damage and controls oxidative activity Regenerates vitamin E Inhibits formation of carcinogenic nitrosamines in the stomach Needed for healthy skin and gums Cofactor in collagen formation (strengthens blood vessel walls, forms scar tissue, provides matrix for bone growth) Thyroxin synthesis Assists with wound healing and resistance to infection Assists with absorption of non-haem iron from plant foods Antioxidant that reduces the risk of some cancers including stomach, mouth, oesophageal, pancreatic and cervical cancers	45 mg	Found in all fruit and vegetables, especially citrus, kiwifruit, berries, guava, pineapple, mango, pawpaw, rockmelon, capsicum, tomatoes, parsley, broccoli, spinach, cabbage

INFORMATION FROM 'BECOMING VEGAN' BY BRENDA DAVIS & VESANTO MELINA, 'COMPLETE FOOD AND NUTRITION COMPANION' BY CATHERINE SAXELBY AND 'UNDERSTANDING NUTRITION' BY ELLIE WHITNEY & SHARON RADY ROLFES

Note: Pregnant and breastfeeding women will have higher requirements than those listed above. This is best checked with your GP, obstetrician or dietitian.

Amounts required for children are often similar or slightly less than adults' requirements. I suggest you refer to information specific to children and check with a paediatrician or dietitian if raising children as vegans.

FAT-SOLUBLE VITAMINS

Fat-soluble vitamins are found in foods that contain fat and remain fairly stable during cooking and processing.

Vitamin	Needed for	Recommended daily intake (RDI)	Vegan food sources
A Occurs as both retinol, found in animal foods and the carotenoid beta-carotene, which is converted by the body into retinol (vitamin A) as needed	Vitamin A is stored in your liver Plays a key role in maintaining healthy vision; maintenance of cornea; protects from night blindness Healthy skin and mucous membranes—keeps the skin in the mouth, respiratory tract and urinary tract moist; protects against harmful bacteria Important for immunity (resistance to infectious diseases) Supports reproduction and normal growth Bone and tooth growth	Women: 700 mcg Men: 900 mcg retinol equivalents Note: toxicity can occur from high doses of retinol *No figures available for beta-carotene	Beta-carotene (vitamin A precursor) is found in orange and green fruit and vegetables e.g. apricots, mango, rockmelon, pawpaw, carrots, sweet potato, pumpkin, spinach, silver beet, parsley, basil, pumpkin, broccoli and chilli *Eat at least one dark green and one orange vegetable or fruit each day to ensure a good carotenoid intake
D (cholecalciferol) Your body synthesises vitamin D with the help of sunlight, from a precursor that the body makes from cholesterol. Although called a vitamin, vitamin D is actually a hormone!	The body requires vitamin D to absorb calcium Part of the bone-making and maintenance team together with calcium, phosphorus, magnesium, fluoride and other compounds and nutrients to make strong, healthy bones and teeth (prevents rickets and osteoporosis) Helps muscles, nerves and immune system work properly Research has shown that vitamin D may be linked to lowering the risk of multiple sclerosis and some cancers	Up to 50: 200 IU 51–70: 400 IU Over 70: 600 IU	The sun! Very small amounts only in food and is mostly fortified Fortified plant milks (e.g. soy) About 10–15 mins/day (or 20 mins every second day) without sunscreen. You will need longer if you have dark skin, aged over 60 and live either above 40° north latitude or below 40° south latitude because synthesis ceases in winter. Practise sun safety and don't go out in the middle of the day

Vitamin	Needed for	Recommended daily intake (RDI)	Vegan food sources
E (tocopherol)	Vitamin E is a powerful antioxidant whose main job is to protect against cell damage by free radicals Strengthens capillary walls Reduces the risk of heart disease by preventing LDL cholesterol oxidation Regulates protein and calcium metabolism Plays a role in maintaining a healthy immune system Protects against cancer	Women: 7 mg Men: 10 mg	Fat-containing foods Wheat germ Wholegrains Nuts, especially almonds and hazelnuts Seeds, especially sunflower seeds Fruit and vegetables, especially dark leafy greens and avocado
K (phylloquinone) There are two forms of vitamin K: vitamin K1 and vitamin K2 Vitamin K2 is made by your body from the vitamin K1 in the food you eat	Essential for blood clotting Vitamin K also helps to build strong bones and protects against hip fractures People who take warfarin, the blood-thinning medication, need to consume the same amount of vitamin K each day Antibiotics can kill the vitamin K2-producing bacteria in the intestine	Women: 60 mcg Men: 70 mcg You need some vitamin K every day for good health	Vitamin K1 is mostly found in plants The main dietary sources of vitamin K are leafy green vegetables such as kale, spinach, Swiss chard, dark lettuce leaves, Asian greens, watercress and parsley, cauliflower and cabbage Vitamin K2 is found in the fermented food natto (and in some meats and cheeses)

INFORMATION FROM 'BECOMING VEGAN' BY BRENDA DAVIS & VESANTO MELINA, 'COMPLETE FOOD AND NUTRITION COMPANION' BY CATHERINE SAXELBY AND 'UNDERSTANDING NUTRITION' BY ELLIE WHITNEY & SHARON RADY ROLFES

MINERALS

Minerals are inorganic elements that originate in the soil. Plants absorb minerals from the soil. Animals get their minerals from the plants or other animals they eat.

Minerals are essential for your body to function optimally, for growth and reproduction. Minerals make up the bony structure of your body and are necessary for chemical reactions, water balance, nerve impulses and muscle contractions.

Major minerals are those present and needed by the body in larger amounts (more than 5 grams—which is about a teaspoon). They include calcium, phosphorus, potassium, sulphur, sodium, chlorine, and magnesium. Trace minerals include iron, zinc, copper, manganese, iodine, fluorine, chromium, selenium, molybdenum and cobalt and are needed in smaller amounts. Despite the amount required, all minerals are vital for optimal health.

Minerals are best obtained from fresh whole food as supplements can be taken in excess which can be toxic. Interactions between minerals, just like with vitamins, can affect their absorption, metabolism and excretion, for example, calcium and iron compete for absorption and high phosphorus levels can limit magnesium absorption. These interactions are usually due to supplement use and are not an issue when eating a variety of whole, fresh food.

Plants can provide all the 21 essential minerals your body needs in adequate amounts for various processes, however the bioavailability, the amount that can be absorbed and used by the body, can vary. Some foods contain binder substances which 'bind' to the mineral throughout the digestive process, preventing its absorption. Examples are oxalates in rhubarb and spinach, and to a lesser extent phytates in legumes and grains whose absorption is more dependent on how the food is prepared. Common preparation methods used in order so that these foods can be consumed usually reduce the effect of phytates. These methods include soaking beans before cooking, leavening bread (leavening occurs when a substance is used to produce fermentation in dough or batter, for example, the process of bread rising through the use of yeast or a sourdough starter), sprouting grains, seeds or legumes, roasting nuts, and fermenting tempeh, miso and natto.

As a vegan, the three main minerals to focus on so you don't fall short are iron, calcium and zinc. I discuss these in detail below. Iodine and sodium also get a small mention. All other minerals I have included in a table for easy reference, but they are generally well obtained from vegan foods.

IRON

Iron is required for growth and development, to make amino acids, hormones, collagen, neurotransmitters, as well as haemoglobin, the central component of red blood cells which transports oxygen around the body, and myoglobin which supplies oxygen to muscles. Iron assists in energy-producing chemical reactions (involved in the electron transport system), plays a role in immunity and in DNA synthesis.

A deficiency can make you feel weak, tired and fatigued and will compromise your immune system, making you more susceptible to catching colds and the flu. Be aware though that an excess of iron mimics symptoms of deficiency, so always diagnose deficiency via a blood test. Check active levels of iron in your blood along with iron stores, called ferritin.

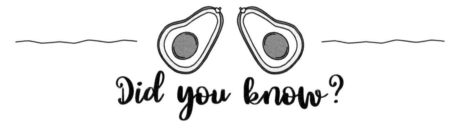

Did you know?

Hemochromatosis refers to too much iron in the body (iron 'overload'). This is usually caused by a genetic disorder which causes the body to absorb extra iron from food.

The body cannot rid itself of extra iron. Over time, excess builds up in major organs. Iron overload damages tissues, especially in the liver, and increases your risk of infections because infections thrive on iron-rich blood.

Chronic fatigue and joint pain are the most common complaints of people with hemochromatosis. Untreated hemochromatosis increases the risk of arthritis, diabetes, heart disease and liver cancer. It's one to be aware of in case you have it.

TYPES OF IRON: HAEM VS NON-HAEM

There are two types of iron. Haem iron is the predominant type found in animal foods such as meat, chicken, fish and offal. Non-haem iron is also found in animal foods, along with eggs, dairy (small amounts) and plant foods such as legumes, nuts, seeds, green leafy vegetables and wholegrains. Haem iron typically has a higher bioavailability, approx. 25 percent, than non-haem iron, approx. 10 percent, but non haem bioavailability depends upon other dietary factors and your body's iron stores.

Non-haem iron absorption is carefully regulated by your gut, according to your need. The body adapts to absorb more iron in those with low iron stores or higher requirements (i.e. during pregnancy) and excretes less. Absorption of non-haem iron is also affected by:

❖ Natural compounds found in plants such as phytates along with associated fibre, oxalates and phosphates can reduce absorption

❖ Tannins found in tea can block absorption. Coffee may also, but to a lesser extent than tea

❖ Excessive calcium–rich foods and supplements if taken at the same meal compete with absorption. Zinc supplements and reflux medications can also reduce absorption

❖ Foods rich in vitamin C (ascorbic acid) can boost absorption. These foods can also override the effects of phytates. Given that all fruit and vegetables contain vitamin C, most vegan meals would naturally include a source of vitamin C, so eating a wide variety of different foods will ensure you get the benefits of vitamin C

❖ Other enhancers of non–haem iron absorption include organic acids such as malic and citric acids commonly found in fruit (citric in citrus) and vegetables, fructose (fruit sugar) and certain amino acids.

How much iron do you need?

Vegan intakes are rich in non-haem iron, which is not absorbed as easily as haem iron, so the recommended iron intake for vegans is greater at 1.8 times that of omnivores.

Age in years	Intake to aim for milligrams (mg) if eating meat /day	Vegan intake (mg) (x 1.8)
Men 19 and older	8	14
Women—19 to menopause	18	32
Post-menopausal women	8	14

INFORMATION FROM NUTRIENT REFERENCE VALUES FOR AUSTRALIA AND NEW ZEALAND AVAILABLE AT HTTPS://WWW.NRV.GOV.AU/NUTRIENTS/IRON|IRON DEFICIENCY

IRON DEFICIENCY DEVELOPS IN STAGES:

1. Stage one (iron deficiency)—iron stores (ferritin) fall below the recommended range.
2. Stage two (iron deficiency)—iron level in blood falls below the recommended range and transferrin (the iron-carrying protein) increases. The higher the transferrin and the lower the iron, the worse this condition.
3. Stage three (iron deficiency anaemia)—the lack of iron affects haemoglobin production and levels fall below the recommended range.

HOW TO AVOID IRON-DEFICIENCY

Make sure you eat iron-rich foods. For vegans these include legumes, soybeans, nuts, seeds, leafy green veggies (apart from spinach and Swiss chard which is also known as silver beet and beetroot greens) and dried fruit.

Tips on meeting your iron needs:

- ❖ include an iron-rich food source at each meal and snack
- ❖ for breakfast, eat oats (topped with nuts and seeds for an added boost) or
- ❖ spread toast with almond or peanut butter for a super-quick option
- ❖ include legumes (beans, lentils, chickpeas, soybeans) in both lunch and dinner (and breakfast if you can)
- ❖ add nuts and/or seeds to your breakfast bowl, salads, stir fries, veggie burgers, baked goods
- ❖ use hummus or nut butters
- ❖ snack on dried fruit, such as dried apricots and figs, along with nuts
- ❖ include leafy green veggies with lunch and/or dinner
- ❖ try foods that are leavened, soaked, fermented or roasted
- ❖ experiment with sprouting seeds because sprouting breaks down phytates, making iron (and zinc) more available and increases vitamin C content (in lentils more than 17 times and in mung beans more than 8 times!)
- ❖ avoid drinking tea with, or close to mealtimes, because tannins can affect iron absorption
- ❖ don't take calcium or zinc supplements with iron-rich foods.

CALCIUM

Calcium is the most abundant mineral in the body.

When most people think of calcium, they immediately think of bones, and for a very good reason as 99 percent of your body's calcium is found in your bones. Calcium combines with other minerals and collagen to give your bones the strength and structure to hold your body upright and provide an attachment for the muscles which allow you to move. Calcium also provides strength and structure in teeth.

The remaining small amount of calcium (1 percent) is distributed in body fluids and soft tissue and is required for the healthy functioning of the heart, muscles, blood cells and nerves. Calcium is essential for blood clotting, muscle relaxation, nerve transmission and regulation of metabolism. It even plays a role in regulating blood pressure.

Your bones act like a calcium 'bank'. If you do not get enough calcium from the food you eat to maintain adequate levels in the blood, the body will 'withdraw' calcium from your 'bone bank' and deposit it into the bloodstream for all those vitally important functions listed above. If your body withdraws more calcium than it deposits over a long period, your bone density (bone strength) will gradually decline and you may be at risk of developing osteoporosis (brittle bones).

Did you know?

While most people focus on getting an adequate calcium intake, weight-bearing exercise is equally as important to assist with building and maintaining strong, healthy bones.

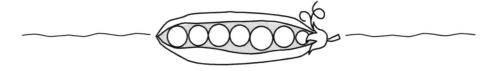

CALCIUM AND AGE

As a child, when you grew, your bones became larger, heavier and denser. Your maximum bone mineral density is achieved by around age 30, with about 45 percent occurring up until 8, another 45 percent from age 8 to 16 and the final 10 percent from age 16 to around 30. After around age 30 to 35, your bone mass starts to decline. How quickly it does so is influenced by what you eat, the medications you take, how much weight-bearing exercise you do and your hormonal balance. When women start to go through menopause and their estrogen levels decline, calcium loss from the bones often increases.

Therefore, it is vital that up until age 30 you maximise your body's ability to accumulate bone strength. A strong start will reduce your chances or delay the risk of developing osteoporosis, where a fall or even a hard knock can result in a fracture or bone breakage.

While an adequate intake of calcium is necessary for bone strength and density, you also need adequate vitamin D levels, as well as adequate intakes of protein, vitamin K, phosphorus, potassium, magnesium and boron.

CALCIUM BALANCE

While consuming enough calcium in your intake and doing an adequate amount of weight-bearing exercise is important for bone strength, ensuring adequate absorption and preventing excess loss from the body is also important.

Calcium can only be absorbed when your vitamin D levels are adequate, so it is important to have your levels checked through a blood test. While sun safety is important to maintain adequate vitamin D levels, if your levels are low, you will need to take a supplement to help increase them initially.

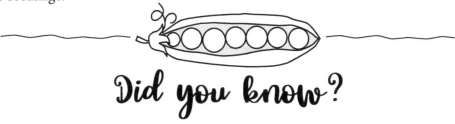

Did you know?

During your lifetime, your body continues to both reabsorb old bone and create new bone. Through this renewal process, your entire skeleton is replaced about every 10 years, though this process slows as you get older. A similar process happens in teeth, but the turnover is not as rapid. Fluoride helps harden and stabilise teeth, preventing mineral loss.

Calcium loss is affected by protein intake. Protein has an acidic effect on the blood which your body neutralises by drawing calcium from the bones. A very high intake of animal protein, which is a concentrated source of both protein and sulphur-containing amino acids, will have a greater effect than plant protein, which is less concentrated in sulphur amino acids. Although a vegan intake is generally more alkaline, high intakes of protein powders (from say soy or pea protein) may contribute to calcium loss. Calcium loss is also increased when there is a very high intake of salt, excessive coffee (caffeine) intake (more than 3 per day) and a high intake of phosphoric acid, which is found in soft drinks like cola.

Certain medicines can increase calcium loss too, for example, long-term use of corticosteroids (for example, prednisone or prednisolone). Long-term use of reflux medications that reduce stomach acid (for example, Somac, Nexium and Zantac) can affect bone health, as can certain medical conditions like overactive parathyroid or adrenal glands, coeliac disease, Crohn's disease and kidney disease. Gastric bypass surgery can affect calcium absorption. A low body weight is also linked to less bone mass and weaker bones.

You absorb calcium more efficiently when a small amount is taken at a time—as calcium dose increases, the percentage absorbed decreases. To maximise calcium absorption, include calcium rich foods across the course of the day rather than all in one meal.

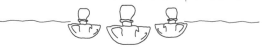

Did you know?

Calcium in dark green leafy vegetables, such as kale, broccoli, and bok choy, is absorbed more easily than calcium from dairy products. These vegetables also include vitamin K, the bone–health superstar!

Calcium absorption from leafy green vegetables is around 50–60 percent whereas absorption from cow's milk is about 30 percent.

SUMMARY OF FACTORS THAT AFFECT CALCIUM BALANCE:

- ❖ You need a 2:1 ratio of calcium to magnesium before calcium can be absorbed
- ❖ Absorption requires adequate hydrochloric acid (HCl) in the stomach and vitamin D in the blood
- ❖ Caffeine and alcohol may inhibit the absorption of calcium in the gut
- ❖ Exercise helps facilitate absorption and regulation of calcium.

BIOAVAILABILITY OF CALCIUM FROM SELECTED FOODS

Percentage absorbed	Food
>50 percent absorbed	Cauliflower, watercress, Brussels sprouts, kale, bok choy, broccoli, calcium fortified foods and beverages*
30 percent absorbed	Milk, cheese, yoghurt, calcium-set tofu, calcium-fortified soymilk*
20 percent absorbed	Almonds, sesame seeds, legumes, sweet potato
<5 percent absorbed	Spinach, Swiss chard, silver beet, rhubarb

INFORMATION FROM 'BECOMING VEGAN' BY
BRENDA DAVIS & VESANTO MELINA

* ABSORPTION VARIES ACCORDING TO THE TYPE
OF CALCIUM USED

VEGAN SOURCES OF CALCIUM:

* ❖ Green leafy vegetables such as kale, Asian greens like bok choy and broccoli
* ❖ Soy products like tofu (if calcium is used to make it—the coagulant is usually magnesium chloride not calcium so check the list of ingredients and the nutrition information panel)
* ❖ Calcium-fortified plant milks such as soy (always check labels)
* ❖ Legumes (lentils, beans and chickpeas)
* ❖ Some dried fruit like figs and apricots
* ❖ Nuts, in particular almonds, almond butter, Brazil nuts and hazelnuts
* ❖ Tahini (sesame seed paste)

NOTES ON VEGAN SOURCES OF CALCIUM

The oxalate level in a plant food is the main determinant of how much calcium can be absorbed.

Low-oxalate, dark leafy greens such as kale, bok choy and broccoli are the best sources of calcium for vegans. In addition to calcium, greens also contain vitamin K, potassium and magnesium, which are all important for bone health.

While spinach, Swiss chard, silver beet and beetroot greens are high in calcium, the calcium isn't well absorbed due to the high content of oxalate, which binds calcium and reduces absorption from the digestive tract.

Soy does not contain a significant amount of calcium. However, calcium is added to many soy-based products, such as calcium-set tofu and soy milk. The calcium in these products is as easily absorbed as it is from dairy. Fortified beverages should be well-shaken to make sure the calcium has not settled to the bottom of the carton.

RECOMMENDATIONS FOR ADEQUATE CALCIUM INTAKE

150 mg of calcium each day is all your bones need to keep up the renewal process, however since only around 30 percent of the calcium present in food is able to be absorbed, you need to aim for an intake of at least 500 mg. Note that absorption is upregulated in children when bones are growing, during pregnancy and is also more efficient in times of inadequate intakes.

The recommended daily intake for this precious mineral takes into consideration bioavailability, nutrient interactions as well as losses in urine and faeces which is dependent upon what you eat—high sodium, high protein will encourage greater loss. Remember that if you do not get enough calcium from food, your body has no choice but to 'rob' (take) from your 'bone bank', increasing your risk of osteoporosis, so it is better to aim higher than lower. Eating a wide variety of food will provide an adequate intake of this essential nutrient without the need to worry about all the little intricacies.

RECOMMENDED DAILY CALCIUM INTAKE

Category	Recommended daily intake (RDI) (mg)
Women 19–50 years old	1000
Women post menopause (>50)	1300
Men 19–70 years old	1000
Men >70	1300

INFORMATION FROM NUTRIENT REFERENCE VALUES FOR AUSTRALIA AND NEW ZEALAND AVAILABLE AT HTTPS://WWW.NRV.GOV.AU/NUTRIENTS/CALCIUM NOTE: CALCIUM REQUIREMENTS INCREASE DURING PREGNANCY AND WHILE BREAST FEEDING.

If considering taking a supplement:

Calcium citrate malate is the form most readily absorbed

Do not exceed 600 mg/day

Do not take with meals as calcium can interfere with iron absorption.

ZINC

While only required in very small amounts, zinc is an incredibly important mineral that supports proteins and enzymes involved in various metabolic processes all throughout your body. Zinc is important for immune function, in particular it aids wound healing and reduces your chance of catching a cold. Very importantly it is required for normal taste and smell. Zinc is part of the hard structure of bones and it assists with respiration, acid-base balance, normal growth (deficiency can contribute to stunted growth in children) and foetal development, sexual maturation and reproduction. Zinc is found in high concentrations in the tissues and fluids of the prostate, sperm and seminal fluid as well as the iris and retina of the eye where it combines with vitamin A to maintain eyesight and delay macular degeneration. It also plays a role in the synthesis, storage and release of the hormone insulin in the pancreas, is part of other pancreatic digestive enzymes and influences thyroid hormone function.

While zinc is not found in high amounts in plant foods, you can absolutely get the amount you need by making sure your daily intake contains plenty of zinc-rich foods. Plant sources of zinc include chickpeas, lentils, beans, tofu, nuts, (especially cashews), and seeds, (especially pumpkin seeds). Zinc is also in wholegrains, however phytates and fibre may reduce bioavailability.

The recommended daily intake of zinc is 8 mg for women and 14 mg for men.

The body actually only needs around 3 mg of zinc each day, but only 10–40 percent of zinc in food is able to be absorbed. Sprouting increases bioavailability of zinc as does the leavening of bread, fermenting of soy foods (tempeh and miso) and roasting nuts breaks down the zinc-phytate complex increasing bioavailability. Calcium supplements can interfere with zinc absorption. Iron supplementation can inhibit zinc absorption and large doses of zinc can inhibit iron absorption and over time (>3 months) may displace copper levels.

Zinc deficiency can cause slow physical growth and delayed sexual maturation in children, poor wound healing, acne, hair loss, reduced ability to taste food properly, lack of appetite, impaired night vision, reduced immune function (increased susceptibility to colds etc.), and dermatitis. Zinc deficiency directly impairs vitamin A metabolism, disturbs thyroid function and your metabolic rate.

Vegan Sources of Calcium, Iron and Zinc

Food	Serving size	Calcium (mg)	Iron (mg)	Zinc (mg)
Almonds, with skin, raw	A handful, 30 g, approx. 23 nuts	75	1.2	1.1
Almond butter, natural	1 tbsp (20 g)	50	0.8	0.7
Amaranth, cooked	½ cup (123 g)	58	2.6	1.1
Apricot, dried	30 g (5 medium halves)	20	1.0	0.2
Baked beans in tomato sauce	½ cup (140 g)	54	1.4	0.7
Black beans, cooked	½ cup (89 g)	51	2.6	0.7
Blackstrap molasses	1 tbsp (28 g)	187	6.7	0.3
Bok choy	½ cup (43 g)	35	0.6	0.2
Brazil nuts	30 g (6–8 nuts)	45	0.7	1.2
Bread, wholemeal with seeds	2 slices (76 g)	72	1.8	1.4
Broccoli, steamed	½ cup (98 g)	30	0.7	0.3
Brown rice, cooked	½ cup (80 g)	10	0.5	0.6
Cannellini beans, cooked	½ cup (130 g)	59	2.0	0.8
Cashews, raw	1 handful, 30 g, approx. 20 medium nuts	10	1.5	1.7
Chia seeds	1 tbsp (14 g)	90	1.1	0.7
Chickpeas, cooked	½ cup (85 g)	39	1.6	0.9
Cocoa powder	1 level tbsp (7 g)	11	1.2	0.6
Edamame	½ cup (73 g)	22	1.3	0.8
Figs, dried	30 g (2 medium)	60	0.4	0.2
Hazelnuts	A handful, 30 g, approx. 21 nuts	26	1.0	0.7
Kale, raw	½ cup chopped (58 g)	20	0.3	0.2
Kidney beans, cooked	½ cup (95 g)	34	2.0	0.6
Lentils, brown, cooked	½ cup (93 g)	19	2.2	0.9
Linseeds	1 tbsp (14 g)	36	0.8	0.6

Food	Serving size	Calcium (mg)	Iron (mg)	Zinc (mg)
Oats, raw	½ cup (40 g)	16	1.4	1.0
Parsley, chopped	2 tbsp (10 g)	19	0.3	0.1
Peanuts	1 handful, 30 g, approx. 40 'nuts'	16	0.7	0.9
Peanut butter	1 tbsp (20 g)	11	0.4	0.5
Peas, cooked	½ cup (73 g)	22	1.3	0.8
Pecans	A handful, 30 g, approx. 10–16 halves	15	0.7	1.2
Pine nuts	30 g, approx. 3 tbsp	3	1.2	1.6
Pistachios	A handful, 30 g, approx. 30+ nuts	27	1.2	0.7
Prunes	30 g, approx. 4–5	16	0.3	0.2
Pumpkin seeds	2 tbsp (30 g)	13	3.0	2.2
Quinoa, cooked	½ cup (96 g)	14	1.2	0.8
Raisins	30 g, approx. ¼ cup	16	0.4	0.1
Silver beet*, cooked	½ cup (58 g)	46	1.5	0.3
Soy beans, cooked	½ cup (95 g)	56	6.4	2.7
Soy milk**	1 cup (250 ml)	296	1.2	0.4
Spinach*, raw	1 cup (45 g)	24	1.4	0.3
Spinach*, steamed	½ cup (60 g)	34	2.0	0.4
Sunflower seeds	2 tbsp (30 g)	23	1.6	1.5
Sweet potato, cooked	½ cup (123 g)	30	0.6	0.6
Tahini*	1 tbsp (20 g)	66	1.0	1.0
Tempeh**	125 g	93	11.5	2.1
Tofu, firm**	½ cup (125 g)	400	3.6	2.1
Tofu, firm**	½ cup (125 g)	400	3.6	2.1
Tofu, soft, silken**	½ cup (125 g)	30	2.2	0.6
Walnuts	A handful, 30 g, approx.15–20 halves	27	0.8	0.8
Watercress, raw	1 cup (33 g)	28	1.0	0.2

DATA FROM FOODWORKS VERSION 8 AND USDA

* Note that spinach (along with Swiss chard, silver beet and beetroot greens) is not a good calcium source as it is high in oxalates which bind the mineral making calcium unavailable. Unhulled tahini may also be high in oxalates.

** Check label for exact amount as brands may vary.

IODINE

In the gut, iodine is converted to iodide, an integral part of the thyroid hormone which regulates your body temperature, metabolic rate, reproduction, growth, blood cell production, nerve and muscle function and more. The hypothalamus in the brain regulates thyroid hormone production through release of TSH (thyroid stimulating hormone) from the pituitary. Iodine deficiency causes low thyroid hormone levels which makes the body produce more TSH. If deficiency persists, high TSH levels promote thyroid tissue growth, causing the gland to enlarge and form a goitre (visible lump in the neck). Excess iodine can also enlarge the thyroid gland and depress thyroid activity.

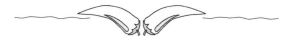

Many people are concerned that certain plants containing goitrogens cause goitre as they block iodine absorption, so they avoid eating cruciferous vegetables such as cabbage and broccoli as well as soy and linseeds. This is a potential problem for those with hypothyroidism, but only when dietary iodine intake is low and an excess of raw goitrogens are consumed, for example, drinking a lot of green smoothies, as cooking dramatically lowers the goitrogenic content of foods. You can avoid these complications by eating a well-varied intake and including a balance of both raw and cooked food.

Iodine deficiency can cause you to feel sluggish and gain weight. Deficiency in pregnancy impairs foetal development and may cause irreversible mental and physical retardation.

Iodine comes mostly from the sea or the soil in which plants are grown. Many people choose to use iodised salt to ensure adequate intake. Regular consumption of seaweed (for example, California rolls and other Japanese foods) can also help you meet your needs.

WHAT ABOUT SALT?

Salt is used to both preserve and flavour food. Salt (sodium chloride) is a combination of sodium and chloride.

A small amount of sodium is necessary for good health as it is required for fluid balance in the body and proper muscle and nerve function. The kidneys regulate your sodium levels.

For years, sodium was held responsible for high blood pressure, however research has shown that salt has a much greater effect on blood pressure than sodium or chloride alone or when sodium is combined with other minerals.

Certain people such as those with hypertension (high blood pressure), diabetes or chronic kidney disease can have a salt sensitivity, meaning they have a greater response to salt. Overweight people may also be more sensitive to the effects of salt, and sensitivity may also increase with age. While reducing salt intake often helps salt-sensitive people to reduce blood pressure, eating an intake abundant with fruit and vegetables (high potassium intake) often has a better outcome.

Salt can be added to your food mindfully and in moderation.
Unless you are under doctor's orders to restrict your use of salt, you should not be afraid to season your food as healthy food should not taste dull or boring.

Did you know?

The majority of sodium in most people's intake, upwards of 75 percent, comes from salt in manufactured food products, particularly bread, processed meat and other processed foods, as well as takeaway and fast foods. Limiting these foods will have the greatest effect on keeping your salt intake low.

Mineral (Major and Trace) Requirements and Food Sources

Mineral	Needed for	Recommended daily intake (RDI)	Vegan food sources
Calcium	Essential for building strong bones and teeth Healthy muscle and nerve function—may relieve pain and cramps Blood clotting Maintaining healthy blood pressure Helps prevent osteoporosis, bowel cancer and kidney stones	1000 mg	Fortified soy milk and tofu Almonds Sesame seeds and tahini Legumes Leafy greens (e.g. kale, broccoli, Asian greens)
Chromium	Normal growth Blood sugar regulation—part of the Glucose Tolerance Factor, which enhances insulin's regulation of blood glucose levels May reduce the risk of type 2 diabetes	Women: 25 mcg Men: 35 mcg	Brewer's yeast Beer Yeast extract Wholegrains and wholegrain products Nuts (especially pecans) Mushrooms Asparagus Prunes Spices—including black pepper
Copper	Facilitates iron absorption and formation of red blood cells Part of several enzymes Aids nervous system functioning Synthesises skin (melanin) and hair pigments Promotes protein metabolism Prevents anaemia	Women: 1.2 mg Men: 1.7 mg High zinc intake can limit absorption	Wholegrains Nuts (especially Brazil nuts and pecans) Seeds Beans Tofu and tempeh Sweet potatoes Bananas Raisins Prunes

Mineral	Needed for	Recommended daily intake (RDI)	Vegan food sources
Fluoride	Increases hardness of tooth enamel, thus decreasing risk of dental caries Mineralisation of bones; helps prevent osteoporosis	Women: 3 mg Men: 4 mg	Fluoridated water Tea Seaweed Some toothpastes
Iodine	An essential part of thyroid hormones Aids thyroid gland function which influences most organ systems Prevents goitre Extremely important in pregnancy Aids brain function	150 mcg	Iodised salt Raw and dried sea vegetables Seaweed
Iron	Key component of haemoglobin in blood which carries oxygen to the tissues Prevents anaemia Part of myoglobin in muscles which makes oxygen available for muscle contraction Participates in the production of brain chemicals (neurotransmitters) such as serotonin and dopamine Component of many enzymes	Women 19–menopause: 32 mg Women post-menopause: 14 mg Men:14 mg	Legumes Dark leafy green vegetables Wholemeal bread Cocoa powder Dried fruit Nuts Seeds
Magnesium	Provides structure for healthy bones and teeth Helps convert food to energy A part of many enzyme systems Supports healthy muscle contraction and nerve function (along with calcium, sodium and potassium) May help relieve muscular pain and cramps May prevent high blood pressure and cardiovascular disease	Women: 320 mg Men: 420 mg	Legumes Tofu Nuts (especially almonds, Brazil nuts) Seeds (especially sunflower seeds) Wholegrains Dates Figs Prunes Bananas Leafy green vegetables

Mineral	Needed for	Recommended daily intake (RDI)	Vegan food sources
Manganese	Activator of (cofactor for) many enzymes	Women: 5 mg Men: 5.5 mg	Nuts Wholegrains Cereals Vegetables Oils
Molybdenum	Cofactor for many enzymes Iron utilisation Alcohol detoxification Metabolism of waste products	45 mcg	Widely distributed in food, especially in vegetables, legumes and grains but dependant on soil content
Phosphorus	Part of the mineral structure of bones and teeth along with calcium Works along with B vitamins Component of proteins and genetic material	1000 mg	Widely distributed in food Excellent sources include: Yeast extract Bran Wheat germ
Potassium	Maintains fluid and electrolyte balance in body Muscle and nerve function Maintains healthy blood pressure—counteracts sodium's adverse effects Depletion can occur following prolonged vomiting or diarrhoea, excessive sweating or excessive intake of processed foods Boiling leaches out potassium so steam your veggies!	Women: 2800 mg Men: 3800 mg	Nuts Yeast extract Bran Wheat germ Fresh fruit (e.g. bananas, cantaloupe/ rockmelon, oranges, peaches, avocado) Vegetables (especially broccoli, Brussels sprouts, green peas, spinach, tomatoes)

Mineral	Needed for	Recommended daily intake (RDI)	Vegan food sources
Selenium	Part of an enzyme that protects the heart and blood cells from oxidative damage Regulates thyroid function for iodine metabolism Immune function Protection from cancer and heart disease	Women: 60 mcg Men: 70 mcg	Brown rice Brazil nuts Wholegrains
Sodium	Controls nerve impulse transmission and muscle contraction along with potassium Helps maintain fluid and electrolyte balance Assists the transport of amino acids and glucose Part of digestive secretions from the pancreas	460–920 mg (approx. 1.2–2.4 g salt or ¼–½ teaspoon	Processed or commercial food products Table, sea and vegetable salts Sauces and stocks Yeast extract Bread (some) Olives Miso Tamari Soy sauce
Zinc	Growth, sexual development and reproduction (concentrated in sperm and prostate) Immune function and wound healing Essential for normal taste, smell and sight Transport of vitamin A Part of insulin and many other enzymes	Women: 8 mg Men: 14 mg	Lentils Chickpeas Beans Tofu Nuts (especially cashews) Seeds (especially pumpkin) Wholegrains Sprouting, fermenting and roasting enhances bioavailability

Information from Becoming Vegan by Brenda Davis & Vesanto Melina, Complete Food and Nutrition Companion by Catherine Saxelby and Understanding Nutrition by Ellie Whitney & Sharon Rady Rolfes

WATER

Water is essential to life.

You can survive without water for only a few days, whereas deficiencies of other nutrients may take anywhere from a few weeks to a few years to develop!

Water is critical to assist the body with all of its vital functions. The body precisely regulates water balance, using several mechanisms, between intake from food and drinks and loss from lungs (through respiration), skin (sweating), kidneys (urine) and in faeces.

Water is an important component of blood, which transports nutrients to cells and collects any waste products, taking them to the kidneys to excrete. Water regulates body temperature, participates in chemical reactions, provides structure to cells and tissues, lubricates joints, internal organs and around the eyes, and maintains blood volume. Water also affects metabolism and may facilitate weight management.

Dehydration occurs when water output exceeds water input. It causes both physical and mental tiredness. Even mild dehydration, as little as 1–2 percent of body weight, can greatly impair cognitive performance: an individual's attentiveness, critical thinking skills and memory. And any athlete can attest to the fact that mild dehydration can negatively impact physical performance.

The minimum daily water intake is 5 x 250 ml glasses for women and 7 glasses for men. More is recommended if you live in a humid environment. Drink up to an extra 1 litre per hour when exercising. The best way to check hydration levels is to look at the colour of your urine. Dark yellow urine is a sign of dehydration. When you are hydrated, your urine should be pale straw, almost clear in colour.

While most people consider water intake their only form of hydration, fruit and vegetables contribute greatly, as do 'fluid' foods like soups, stews and other 'wet' dishes along with plant milks, juices and smoothies.

Did you know?

Depending on body composition, water comprises about 60 percent of an adult's body weight.
Lean body tissue, which includes muscles, organs and bones, is around 75 percent water whereas water in fat tissue varies between 10–25 percent.

Putting it all together: food groups

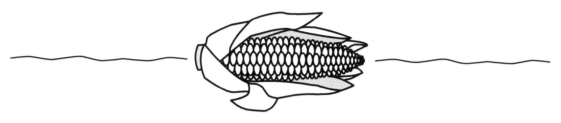

THE ADULT VEGAN FOOD GROUP GUIDE

How to get all the nutrition you need in your daily meals.

Now that you understand macro- and micronutrients, how do you apply this information to your daily meals? You can't simply eat a bowl of folate or protein!

To meet your nutritional requirements, you need to include a wide variety of different foods each day. This food group guide can assist you to get the most from your meals.

The guide is based on the Australian Dietary Guidelines but has been slightly adapted for vegans. It is also aligned with the food guide from Becoming vegan: The complete guide to adopting a healthy plant-based diet by Davis and Melina (see References).

Daily serving sizes will vary according to your age, your activity level and your height.

Note that some food groups overlap. In particular, the beans/legumes group overlaps with the calcium group. The calcium category overlaps slightly with the vegetable group.

You will notice that the calcium category has 6 to 8 serves listed, which may seem a lot. That is because the serving size is small as it is based on the amount a person would typically consume.

Limit extra foods such as high-fat, sugary, salty foods and drinks, for example, confectionary, soft drinks, alcohol, cakes, biscuits, chocolate and fried take-away foods. These are not 'everyday foods'.

Drink 6 to 8 glasses of water every day.

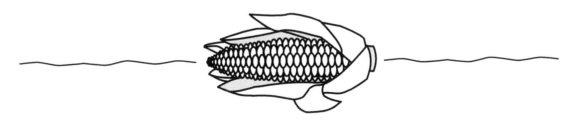

Food group	Serves/day	Serving size
Vegetables	Women: min. 5 Men <70: min. 6 Men >70: min. 5	Seasonal is best. Choose a wide variety of different colours ½ cup cooked green or orange vegetables (e.g. broccoli, spinach, carrots or pumpkin) 1 medium tomato 1 cup green leafy or raw salad vegetables ½ cup sweet corn ½ medium potato or other starchy vegetables (sweet potato, taro or cassava)
Fruit	2	Seasonal is best. Choose a wide variety of different colours 1 medium sized apple, banana, orange or pear 2 small apricots, kiwifruit or plums 1 cup diced or canned fruit (no added sugar) 125 ml (½ cup) fruit juice (no added sugar) (only occasionally) 30 g dried fruit (e.g. 4 dried apricot halves, 1½ tbsp of sultanas)
Beans/legumes and legume alternatives	2–3	1 cup (150 g) cooked or canned legumes/beans (e.g. lentils, chickpeas or split peas) (preferably with no added salt) 170 g tofu 2 cups soymilk 30 g nuts, seeds, peanut or almond butter, tahini or other 100 percent nut or seed butters. This gives approximately the same amount of energy as the other foods in this group but will provide less protein, iron or zinc
Calcium rich foods Note that some of these foods double as serves from the beans, vegetable or fruit group	6–8	½ cup (125 ml) soy, almond or other plant-based milk with at least 100 mg of calcium per 100 ml 50 g firm tofu (check the label as calcium levels vary) 50 grams almonds or almond butter 1 cup cooked or 2 cups raw calcium-rich greens (kale, broccoli, okra, Asian greens) 1 cup calcium-rich beans (cannellini, black beans) 2 teaspoons blackstrap molasses 3 dried figs
Grains	3–6	Choose wholegrain 1 slice (40 g) bread ½ cup cooked rice, pasta, noodles, barley, buckwheat, semolina, polenta, bulgur or quinoa ½ cup cooked porridge ⅔ cup (30 g) breakfast cereal; ¼ cup (30 g) muesli
Essential fatty acids (EFAs)	1–2	1 tsp flaxseed oil 30 g walnuts 1 tbsp ground or whole linseeds or chia seeds
Vitamin B12	2.4 mcg	Fortified foods Supplement

INFORMATION ADAPTED FROM AUSTRALIAN DIETARY GUIDELINES AND 'BECOMING VEGAN' BY AMERICAN DIETITIANS BRENDA DAVIS AND VESANTO MELINA

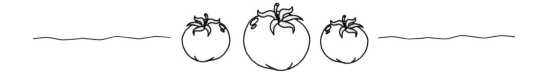

How To Check Your Intake

FOOD DIARY

If you want to track your intake to make sure it includes all that you need, use this chart to monitor what you eat over the week. Take note of your serving sizes and mark the corresponding check boxes for the food group. This chart can help you easily identify if you are eating too much from one group and not enough from another. See examples of how to do this on the following pages.

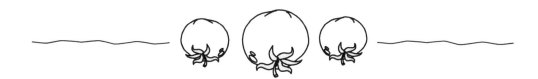

MONDAY

Vegetable ☐☐☐☐☐☐
Fruit ☐☐
Beans/legumes ☐☐☐
Calcium ☐☐☐☐☐☐☐
Grains ☐☐☐☐☐☐
EFAs ☐☐
Vitamin B12 ☐

TUESDAY

Vegetable ☐☐☐☐☐☐
Fruit ☐☐
Beans/legumes ☐☐☐
Calcium ☐☐☐☐☐☐☐
Grains ☐☐☐☐☐☐
EFAs ☐☐
Vitamin B12 ☐

WEDNESDAY

Vegetable ☐☐☐☐☐☐
Fruit ☐☐
Beans/legumes ☐☐☐
Calcium ☐☐☐☐☐☐☐
Grains ☐☐☐☐☐☐
EFAs ☐☐
Vitamin B12 ☐

THURSDAY

Vegetable ☐☐☐☐☐☐
Fruit ☐☐
Beans/legumes ☐☐☐
Calcium ☐☐☐☐☐☐☐
Grains ☐☐☐☐☐☐
EFAs ☐☐
Vitamin B12 ☐

FRIDAY

Vegetable ☐☐☐☐☐☐
Fruit ☐☐
Beans/legumes ☐☐☐
Calcium ☐☐☐☐☐☐☐
Grains ☐☐☐☐☐☐
EFAs ☐☐
Vitamin B12 ☐

SATURDAY

Vegetable ☐☐☐☐☐☐
Fruit ☐☐
Beans/legumes ☐☐☐
Calcium ☐☐☐☐☐☐☐
Grains ☐☐☐☐☐☐
EFAs ☐☐
Vitamin B12 ☐

SUNDAY

Vegetable ☐☐☐☐☐☐
Fruit ☐☐
Beans/legumes ☐☐☐
Calcium ☐☐☐☐☐☐☐
Grains ☐☐☐☐☐☐
EFAs ☐☐
Vitamin B12 ☐

WHAT DO I NEED MORE OF?

☐
☐
☐
☐
☐
☐
☐

In order to reach my daily targets I need to:

_____

_____

_____

_____

I can do that if I:

_____

_____

_____

_____

_____

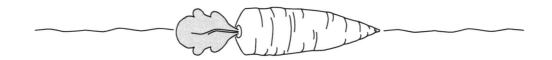

Example One

A TYPICAL DAY'S INTAKE

BREAKFAST

❖ Bircher muesli with nuts, seeds and fruit

LUNCH

❖ Chickpea falafels with salad

DINNER

❖ Lentil Bolognese on wholemeal pasta with a side of broccoli

SNACKS

❖ Fresh fruit
❖ Dried fruit with nuts

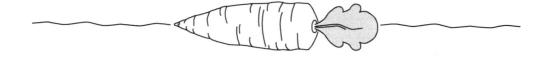

Food group	Breakfast	Lunch	Dinner	Snack	Servings
Vegetables		2 cups salad (2 serves)	In Bolognese – onion, mushrooms, eggplant, tomato (approx. 1½ cups) + ½ cup broccoli = 4 serves		6 Goal 5–6
Fruit	½ apple + ¼ cup berries (¾ serve)			Banana (1 serve) 3 figs (1 serve) = 2 serves	2¾ Goal 2
Beans/ legumes	1 cup soy milk = ½ serve	1 cup chickpeas (1 serve) + 30 g almonds (1 serve) = 2 serves	1 cup lentils (1 serve)		3½ Goal 2–3
Calcium	2 teaspoon blackstrap molasses (1 serve) 1 cup soymilk (2 serves) = 3 serves	1 cup chickpeas (½ serve) 30 g almonds (½ serve) = 1 serve	½ cup broccoli (½serve)	3 dried figs (1 serve) 20g almonds (½ serve) = 1½ serves	6 Goal 6–8
Grains	1/3 cup oats (1½ serves)		1 cup cooked pasta (2 serves)		3½ Goal 3–6
EFAs	1 tablespoon ground linseeds (1 serve) + 30 g walnuts (1 serve) = 2 serves	1 teaspoon flaxseed oil in salad dressing (1 serve)			3 Goal 1–2
Vitamin B12			1 tablespoon fortified nutritional yeast		1 Goal 2.4 mcg

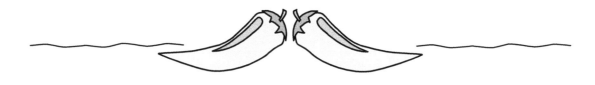

Example Two

A TYPICAL DAY'S INTAKE

BREAKFAST

❖ Toast with almond butter
❖ + B12 supplement

LUNCH

❖ Pumpkin leek and red lentil soup
❖ An apple and a handful of walnuts

DINNER

❖ Bean chilli on quinoa with sunflower seed
sour 'cream' and salad

SNACKS

❖ Energy balls
❖ Smoothie

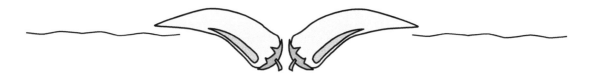

Food group	Breakfast	Lunch	Dinner	Snack	Servings
Vegetables		Cooked pumpkin and leek (approx. 2 cups) = 2 serves	Onion, mushrooms, tomato (approx. 1½ cups cooked) + ½ cup broccoli = 4 serves		6 Goal 5–6
Fruit		Apple (1 serve)		Smoothie— Banana (1 serve) Energy balls Dried fruit (1 serve) = 2 serves	3 Goal 2
Beans/ legumes		½ cup lentils (½ serve) 30 g walnuts (1 serve) = 2 serves	½ cup red kidney beans (½ serve) ½ cup black beans (½ serve) = 1 serve	30g almonds (1 serve) 1 cup soy milk = ½ serve	4 Goal 2–3
Calcium	2 tbsp almond butter (1 serve)	1 cup lentils (¼ serve)	1 cup cooked kale (1 serve) + ½ cup red kidney beans (½ serve) + ½ cup black beans (½ serve) + 2 tablespoon sunflower seed 'cream' (½ serve) = 2½ serves	Energy balls have 3 dried figs (1 serve) + 30 g almonds (½ serve) Smoothie with 1 cup soy milk (1 serve) = 3 serves	6 ¼ Goal 6–8
Grains	2 slices grain bread (2 serves)		1 cup cooked quinoa (2 serves)		4 Goal 3–6
EFAs		30 g walnuts (1 serve)		Smoothie with 1 tablespoon ground linseeds (1 serve)	2 Goal 1–2
Vitamin B12	Supplement				1 Goal 2.4 mcg

Putting it all together: What to eat at each meal

BREAKFAST

Breakfast is key to starting the day in a balanced way and it makes an important contribution towards your daily nutrient intake. Eating a healthy, filling breakfast will help keep blood sugar levels stable and prevent you craving unhealthy foods later in the day.

BREAKFAST NEEDS TO INCLUDE:

- ❖ Low GI, high fibre carbohydrate
- ❖ Plant protein source
- ❖ Healthy fat
- ❖ Fruit and/or vegetables where you can

BREAKFAST SUGGESTIONS

Super-fast Breakfast Ideas

- ❖ Smoothie made with calcium-fortified plant milk with mixed fruit (mango, berries, banana), ground linseeds or chia seeds and a tablespoon of oats
- ❖ Bircher muesli that includes oats, seeds, nuts, fruit and nut or soymilk (make night before and can take with you if needed)
- ❖ Homemade granola, based on oats or buckwheat, seeds and nuts served with nut or soymilk or dairy-free yoghurt and fruit
- ❖ Toast with natural peanut butter, almond butter, tahini or other 100 percent nut or seed butters
- ❖ Toast with hummus, tomato and seeds
- ❖ Avocado, tomato and seeds (sunflower, linseeds etc.) on wholegrain toast
- ❖ Baked beans (tinned) on toast or just as they are!
- ❖ Homemade healthy muesli bar or muffin that contains grains, fruit, nuts and/or seeds

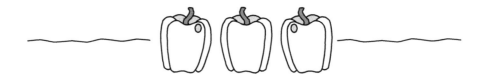

LEISURELY BREAKFAST OPTIONS

- ❖ Tofu scramble with wholegrain toast and vegetables such as sautéed spinach and mushrooms
- ❖ Porridge—rolled or steel cut oats cooked with calcium-fortified plant milk like soy milk, topped with fruit, nuts and seeds
- ❖ Homemade baked beans with spinach and mushrooms
- ❖ Breakfast burrito filled with whole or refried beans and veggies
- ❖ Breakfast bowl with baked beans, avocado, other baked or pan-fried veggies, tofu, etc.
- ❖ Healthy pancakes with fruit and plant-based yoghurt or cashew 'cream'
- ❖ Fruit compote with plant-based yoghurt or cashew 'cream'

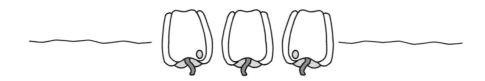

LUNCH AND DINNER

I've included lunch and dinner together here as they require the same components. The only difference will be the portion sizes, depending on which meal you decide is your main one and of course, how hungry you are. Both lunch and dinner need to include:

PROTEIN

- ❖ Legumes
- ❖ Tofu
- ❖ Nuts
- ❖ Seeds

LOW GI CARBOHYDRATE

- ❖ Legumes;
- ❖ Grains (rice, quinoa, barley);
- ❖ Starchy veggies (potatoes, sweet potato, corn); OR
- ❖ Wholegrain or
- ❖ Sourdough bread

NON-STARCHY VEGETABLES OR SALAD

- ❖ Alfalfa and other sprouts,
- ❖ Artichoke, Asian Greens, Asparagus,
- ❖ Baby Squash,
- ❖ Beetroot, Beans, Broccoli,
- ❖ Brussels Sprouts,
- ❖ Cabbage, Capsicum,
- ❖ Carrots, Cauliflower, Celery,
- ❖ Choko, Cucumber,
- ❖ Eggplant, Endive/Fennel,
- ❖ Green Beans, Leeks,
- ❖ Lettuce, Marrow, Mushrooms, Okra, Onion, Parsnip Peas/Snow Peas Pumpkin, Radish, Shallots,
- ❖ Silverbeet, Snake Beans,
- ❖ Spinach, Swede,
- ❖ Tomato/Tomato Paste/Purée,
- ❖ Turnip, Watercress,
- ❖ Zucchini/Squash

SMALLER MEAL IDEAS

❖ Mixed bean salad with spinach leaves, tomato and avocado with an extra virgin olive oil or flaxseed oil-based vinaigrette
❖ Sandwich (2 slices bread) with hummus, avocado, sprouts and salad
❖ Mixed salad leaves with quinoa, chickpeas, veggies, mixed seeds and a tahini and lemon dressing
❖ Veggie burger with salad
❖ Pumpkin, leek and red lentil soup or other soups with veggies and legumes
❖ Refried bean burrito or wrap with salad

LARGER MEAL IDEAS

❖ Vegan shepherd's pie made with lentils and vegetables and topped with sweet potato mash
❖ Tofu and vegetable stir-fry with brown rice and quinoa mix, sprinkled with toasted sesame seeds
❖ Pulse (pasta made from 100 percent legumes) or wholemeal pasta and lentil bolognaise topped with nutritional yeast or cashew 'cheese' with steamed greens or salad
❖ Chickpea, pumpkin and spinach curry with brown rice and cashews
❖ A big bowl of veggie and bean chilli topped with avocado and coriander

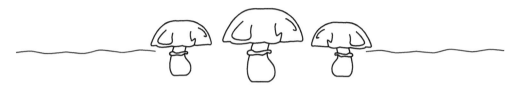

SNACKS

Snacks can make an important contribution towards your daily nutrient intake and help you meet all of your nutritional needs so choose carefully.

Whether you snack, how often you snack and how much you eat depends on your age, activity levels and how much you consume at mealtimes. Here are some examples:

- ❖ Wholegrain or seedy crackers with natural 100 percent nut or seed butter or healthy dips (for example, hummus)
- ❖ Cut up veggies with hummus or other healthy dips
- ❖ Fresh fruit and nuts
- ❖ Dried figs, apricots and prunes with nuts or seeds
- ❖ Smoothies
- ❖ Soup with legumes
- ❖ Energy balls—usually with a base of dried fruit and nuts or seeds
- ❖ Homemade healthy biscuits, cakes, slices (see my website for ideas)

Menu Plans with analysis for Calcium, Iron and Zinc

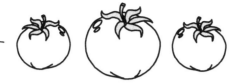

Menu One

BREAKFAST

❖ Porridge with linseeds, pumpkin seeds,
dried figs, made with soymilk
❖ Coffee made with soymilk

MORNING SNACK

❖ Handful of cashews
❖ 4 dried apricots

LUNCH

❖ Salad with chickpeas, edamame and seeds
—liquid gold dressing
❖ 2 slices wholegrain bread spread with tahini

AFTERNOON SNACK

❖ Hommus with carrot sticks and
seedy crackers (recipe from healthyhomecafe.com)

DINNER

❖ Stir fry tofu with veggies and quinoa

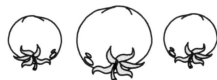

	Calcium (g)	Iron (mg)	Zinc (mg)
BREAKFAST			
½ cup rolled oats	16	1.4	1.0
1 tablespoon linseeds	36	0.8	0.6
1 tablespoon pumpkin seeds	5	1.2	0.9
2 dried figs	76	0.5	0.2
1 cup soy milk	309	1.2	0.4
SNACK			
Coffee with soy milk (regular size)	209	1.1	0.4
Handful of cashews (36 grams)	12	1.8	2.0
4 dried apricots (20 grams)	13	0.9	0.2
LUNCH			
2 cups salad leaves	89	1.4	0.4
½ cup cooked chickpeas	39	1.6	0.9
¼ avocado, 6 cherry tomatoes	7	0.3	0.2
¼ cup edamame	25	0.9	0.6
1 tablespoon sunflower seeds	4	0.2	0.2
1 tablespoon pumpkin seeds	5	1.2	0.9
1 tablespoon flaked almonds	25	0.4	0.4
1 tablespoon liquid gold dressing	10	0.1	0.0
2 slices wholegrain bread	106	1.7	1.3
2 tablespoons tahini	132	2.0	2.2
SNACK			
3 tablespoons hommus	39	1.0	0.8
1 carrot	39	0.4	0.3
8 seedy crackers*	69	2.3	1.8
DINNER			
100 grams bok choy	83	1.4	0.4
½ small red capsicum	5	0.3	0.2
1 small carrot	39	0.4	0.3
½ zucchini, ¼ red onion, 1 clove garlic	15	0.4	0.2
¼ cup edamame	25	0.9	0.6
150 grams firm tofu	480	4.4	2.6
1 cup cooked quinoa	28	3.7	2.5
TOTAL	**1940**	**33.9**	**22.5**
RDI—Women 19–50	1000	32.0	8.0
RDI—Women 50+	1300	14.0	8.0
RDI—Men 19–70	1000	14.0	14.0
RDI—Men 70+	1300	14.0	14.0

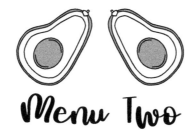

Menu Two

BREAKFAST

- ❖ Baked Beans (tinned) with cashew cheese and sautéed mushrooms on 1 slice toast
- ❖ Coffee with soymilk

LUNCH

- ❖ Pumpkin, black bean and coriander soup (recipe from healthyhomecafe.com)
- ❖ 1 slice bread spread with avocado

SNACKS

- ❖ Seedy crackers with peanut butter
- ❖ 1 orange
- ❖ Handful of almonds
- ❖ 3 tahini cookies (recipe from healthyhomecafe.com)

DINNER

- ❖ Super-fast chilli (recipe from healthyhomecafe.com)
- ❖ Served on quinoa with fresh steamed greens

BREAKFAST	Calcium (g)	Iron (mg)	Zinc (mg)
11/3 cups baked beans, tinned	142	3.7	1.9
1 slice wholegrain bread	53	0.9	0.7
2 large mushrooms	5	0.7	0.1
2 tablespoons cashew cheese (45 grams)	7	1.0	1.1
1 teaspoon extra virgin olive oil	0	0.0	0.0
Flat white coffee with soymilk	185	1.2	0.4
SNACK			
8 seedy crackers	69	2.3	1.8
2 tablespoons peanut butter	22	0.9	1.4
LUNCH			
Pumpkin soup with ½ onion, 250 grams pumpkin, 1 cup stock	74	0.9	0.5
½ cup black beans, tinned	50	1.8	0.8
2 tablespoons fresh coriander	8	0.7	0.0
1 slice wholegrain bread	53	0.9	0.7
¼ small avocado	3	0.2	0.1
SNACK			
1 orange	63	0.9	0.4
2 handfuls of almonds (60 grams)	150	2.4	2.2
3 figs	114	0.8	0.3
3 tahini biscuits*	44	1.4	1.8
DINNER			
Chilli*	129	4.8	2.0
2 tablespoons coriander	8	0.6	0.0
1 cup cooked quinoa	28	3.7	2.5
4 stalks broccolini	36	0.9	0.5
½ cup steamed green beans	21	0.8	0.6
TOTAL	1268	31.5	19.8
RDI—Women 19-50	1000	32.0	8.0
RDI—Women 50+	1300	14.0	8.0
RDI—Men 19-70	1000	14.0	14.0
RDI—Men 70+	1300	14.0	14.0

Menu Three

BREAKFAST

- ❖ Scrambled tofu
- ❖ 2 slices wholegrain toast spread with avocado

SNACKS

- ❖ 2 kiwi fruit
- ❖ Handful of walnuts
- ❖ 3 Medjool dates
- ❖ 2 peanut butter and chickpea energy balls
  (recipe from healthyhomecafe.com)

LUNCH

- ❖ 2 lentil burger patties
  (recipe from healthyhomecafe.com)
- ❖ On a wholegrain bun spread with tahini and salad

DINNER

- ❖ Quick coconut and chickpea curry (recipe from
  healthyhomecafe.com)
- ❖ Served on quinoa with fresh steamed greens

Nutritional requirements are individual and change in different
life stages as well. For a personally tailored vegan meal plan, see an
accredited practising dietitian.

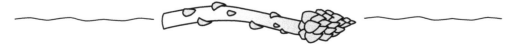

BREAKFAST	Calcium (g)	Iron (mg)	Zinc (mg)
150 grams firm tofu	480	2.7	0.8
1 tablespoon soymilk	25	0.1	0
1 teaspoon turmeric	22	1.0	0.1
1 medium tomato	14	0.4	0.5
1 tablespoon pumpkin seeds	5	1.2	0.9
2 slices wholegrain bread	107	1.7	1.3
¼ avocado	5	0.2	0.2
Café latte—regular with soymilk (280 ml)	209	1.1	0.4
SNACKS			
2 kiwi fruit	41	0.6	0.2
1 handful walnuts (30 grams)	27	0.8	0.8
3 Medjool dates	32	1.8	0.4
LUNCH			
2 lentil burger patties*	75	4.1	2.4
1 wholemeal bread roll	62	1.7	0.8
1 tablespoon tahini	66	1.0	1.1
1 cup salad leaves	44	0.7	0.2
½ medium tomato	4	0.1	0.2
SNACK			
2 peanut butter and chickpea energy balls*	24	1.0	0.9
DINNER			
Quick chickpea and coconut curry*	145	6.5	2.3
1 cup quinoa	28	3.7	2.5
4 stalks broccolini	45	0.9	0.5
½ cup steamed green beans	21	0.8	0.6
TOTAL	1481	32.1	17.1
RDI—Women 19–50	1000	32.0	8.0
RDI—Women 50+	1300	14.0	8.0
RDI—Men 19–70	1000	14.0	14.0
RDI—Men 70+	1300	14.0	14.0

FOODWORKS VERSION 8 WAS USED TO CALCULATE THE NUTRITIONAL ANALYSIS

*RECIPES FROM HEALTHYHOMECAFE.COM

Notes

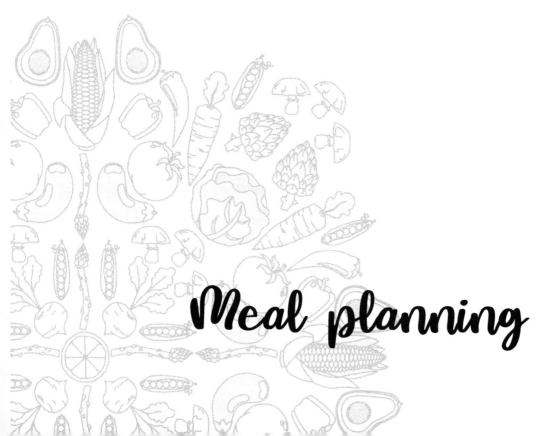

Meal planning

HOW TO EAT WELL

If you fail to plan, you are planning to fail!

The key to eating well is in the planning. Plan what you are going to eat for the week, then on the weekend or when you have more time, you can shop and prepare for the days ahead.

Using a format like this can help or you can just plan dinners for Monday to Thursday when starting out and make extra to take for lunch the following day.

Meal	Monday	Tuesday	Wednesday	Thursday	Friday
Breakfast					
Lunch					
Dinner					
Snacks (optional)					

GUIDELINES TO HELP WITH PLANNING:

1. Start by choosing quick, yummy, familiar recipes
2. Make a shopping list from your plan and stick to it
3. Pre-prepare when you have time, for example, on the weekend
4. Batch cook and freeze
5. Cook once, eat 2 or 3 times

Once you are an efficient planner, you can then experiment with new foods and recipes. This is best done on the weekend or when you have more time rather than during the week, especially if you tend to always be time poor. If they are a hit and quick and easy to prepare, once you are familiar with these new foods/recipes, you can include them during your busy week.

Some of my clients also love to have a format to follow when they first start out with planning. Here is an example of a format:

- ❖ Monday > veggie burgers (make on the weekend)
- ❖ Tuesday > tacos, wraps or pasta
- ❖ Wednesday > stir-fry night
- ❖ Thursday > something from the freezer like Bolognese, curry, chilli, a hearty soup or other 'wet' dish or a 10-minute meal
- ❖ Friday > leftovers, superfast meal or healthy take-away

Weekly Shopping List

LEGUMES

GRAINS

NUTS AND SEEDS

FRUIT AND VEG

GROCERIES

OTHER

SPRING/SUMMER MEAL PLANS

WEEK ONE

Meal	Monday	Tuesday	Wednesday	Thursday	Friday
Breakfast	Granola with nuts, seeds and berries	Toast with avocado and seeds	Granola with nuts, seeds and fruit	Toast with 100 percent nut or seed butter	Toast with avocado and seeds
Lunch	Mixed bean salad with spinach leaves and avocado on toast	Leftover lentil burgers with salad	Leftover chilli	Leftover chickpea burgers	Leftover tacos or sandwich with hummus, avocado, sprouts and salad
Dinner	Lentil and cashew burgers with salad	Fast fabulous bean chilli with lime and avocado	Chickpea burgers with sprouted lentil salad	Black bean soft tacos with guacamole and slaw	Stir-fry with tofu, brown rice and cashews

SNACK SUGGESTIONS: FRESH SEASONAL FRUIT, NUTS, HEALTHY DIPS WITH CUT UP VEGGIES OR SEEDY CRACKERS

MAKE AHEAD NOTES - WEEKEND MEAL PREP

❖ Make granola and store in an airtight jar
❖ Make lentil and cashew burger mix and store in the fridge
❖ Make chickpea burger mix and store in the fridge
❖ Start the process of sprouting lentils over the weekend
❖ Make salad dressings and store in the fridge

SPRING/SUMMER MEAL PLANS

WEEK TWO

Meal	Monday	Tuesday	Wednesday	Thursday	Friday
Breakfast	Bircher muesli with nuts and seeds	Toast with 100 percent nut or seed butter	Bircher muesli with nuts and seeds	Toast with hummus, tomato and seeds	Seasonal fruit with plant-based yoghurt, nuts and seeds
Lunch	Super Greens Salad with Quinoa, Chickpeas, Nuts and Seeds	Leftover Mushroom Tart and Salad	Leftover Tofu Burgers	Leftover Falafels and Salad	Leftover Pesto Pasta Salad
Dinner	Mushroom Lentil and Walnut Tart with Simple Spinach Salad	Tofu Burgers with Avocado and Salad	Falafels with Lemony Tahini Sauce and Salad	Pesto Pasta Salad	Tofu Greens and Cashew Stir-fry with Quinoa

SNACK SUGGESTIONS: FRESH SEASONAL FRUIT, NUTS, HEALTHY DIPS WITH CUT UP VEGGIES OR SEEDY CRACKERS

MAKE AHEAD NOTES - WEEKEND MEAL PREP

- ❖ Make Bircher muesli and store in the fridge
- ❖ Make lentil and walnut tart and store in the fridge
- ❖ Make salad dressings and pesto and store in the fridge
- ❖ Make falafel mix on the weekend and store in the fridge

AUTUMN/WINTER MEAL PLANS

WEEK ONE

Meal	Monday	Tuesday	Wednesday	Thursday	Friday
Breakfast	Porridge with nuts and seeds	Toast with 100 percent nut butter	Chai spiced porridge	Toast with 100 percent nut or seed butter	Baked beans
Lunch	Cauliflower Red Lentil and Coconut Soup with Toast	Roasted Pumpkin Soup with Black Beans and Coriander	Leftover chilli or Pumpkin Soup	Leftover Chickpea Curry	Leftover Lentil Bolognese
Dinner	Stir-fry Tofu with Veggies, Brown Rice/ Quinoa Mix and Cashews	Chilli Sin Carne with Avocado and Coriander on Brown Rice or Quinoa	Quick Coconut and Chickpea Curry with Quinoa	Lentil Bolognese on Wholemeal or Pulse Pasta	Satay Tofu with greens

SNACK SUGGESTIONS: ENERGY BALLS, SEEDY CRACKERS WITH NUT BUTTER OR HUMMUS, APRICOT, MACADAMIA, DATE AND GINGER COOKIES, HOMEMADE MUESLI BAR

MAKE AHEAD NOTES -WEEKEND MEAL PREP

❖ Make cauliflower and pumpkin soups. Store in the fridge and freeze any leftovers that you won't be eating this week
❖ Make a large batch of Lentil bolognese and freeze in meal-sized portions
❖ Cook quinoa on the weekend and freeze in meal-sized portions
❖ Make Quick coconut chickpea curry and store in the fridge
❖ Make snacks if including

AUTUMN WINTER MEAL PLANS

WEEK TWO

Meal	Monday	Tuesday	Wednesday	Thursday	Friday
Breakfast	Porridge with Nuts and Seeds	Carrot Quinoa and Seed Loaf with Avocado or Nut/Seed Butter	Sticky Date Porridge	Baked Beans on Toast or Carrot Quinoa and Seed Loaf	Healthy muffin or muesli bars
Lunch	Barley and Chickpea Salad with Tahini Dressing	Pumpkin Leek and Red Lentil Soup	Leftover Dhal and Roti	Leftover Chilli	Leftover Minestrone
Dinner	Carrot and Red Lentil Soup with Seedy Soda Bread Rolls	Mushroom, Pea and Cashew Curry with Dhal and Roti	Black Bean Chilli on Polenta	Minestrone	Super-fast Nachos with Steamed Greens or Salad

SNACK SUGGESTIONS: PEANUT BUTTER AND CHICKPEA PROTEIN BALLS, SEEDY APRICOT AND TAHINI BALLS, NUT BARS

MAKE AHEAD NOTES - WEEKEND MEAL PREP

❖ Make carrot soup and minestrone. freeze minestrone and any leftover carrot soup that you won't be eating this week
❖ Make mushroom curry and dhal and store in the fridge
❖ Make black bean chilli and store in the fridge
❖ Make snacks if including any

Notes

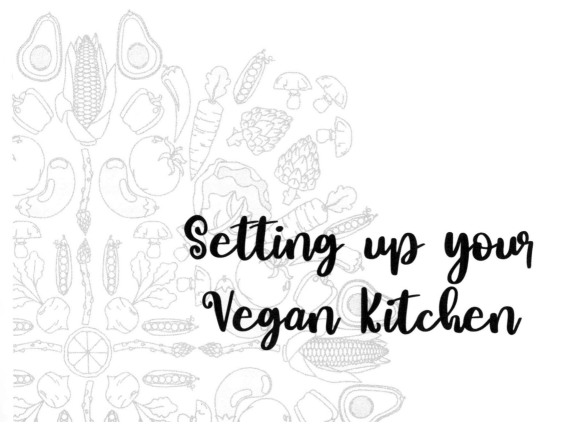

Setting up your Vegan Kitchen

VEGAN PANTRY ESSENTIALS

Having a good supply of ingredients on hand and ready to use in your pantry will help streamline your cooking and allow you to whip up quick, tasty meals most nights of the week. Here is a list of my favourite pantry items:

TINS

- Baked beans
- Refried beans
- Legumes: choose a wide variety such as lentils, black beans, cannellini beans, 4 or 5-bean mix, chickpeas
- Tomatoes: diced, whole
- Coconut milk

JARS

- Pasta sauce
- Tomato paste
- Peanut butter and any other 100 percent nut butters such as almond, cashew and blends like almond, Brazil and cashew
- Tahini or other 100 percent seed butters
- Mustard
- Chutney
- Relish

BOTTLES

- Extra virgin olive oil
- Flaxseed oil (store in fridge)
- Toasted sesame oil
- Balsamic vinegar
- Sweet chilli sauce
- Tomato sauce
- Soy sauce or tamari (gluten free, lower salt soy)
- Worcestershire sauce (check for those without anchovies in ingredients)
- Maple syrup, other sweeteners

DRIED HERBS AND SPICES

- Oregano
- Rosemary
- Curry powder
- Mixed spice blends such as Mexican or Moroccan
- Smoked and/or sweet paprika
- Turmeric
- Cumin
- Coriander
- Cinnamon
- Nutmeg
- Salt
- Pepper

DRY GOODS

- Red lentils
- Other lentils, beans and chickpeas
- Pasta, for example, San Remo Pulse Pasta made from legumes (it's delicious!)
- Brown rice
- Quinoa
- Barley
- Oats
- Other wholegrains such as buckwheat, millet, bulgur
- Nuts (best kept in the fridge)
- Seeds (again, I prefer to store in fridge)
- Flour: wholemeal, besan (chickpea), coconut, etc.

OTHERS

- Liquid stock or stock powder/cubes (Massel is vegan)
- Miso (store in fridge after opening)

SETTING UP YOUR KITCHEN

When it comes to eating healthily, you will need to prepare and cook the majority of your food. So it helps to have a well set up kitchen to make cooking easier and more enjoyable. In this section I have included a list of my favourite kitchen equipment along with tips on how best to cook and prepare delicious, healthy food.

KITCHEN ESSENTIALS

Here I have included a list of what I believe to be the 15 most important items you need in your kitchen. The list starts off with those items that are a lot more important, through to those that are nice to have.

1. KNIVES

Invest in a set of quality knives that you keep sharp. My favourite knives are Global as they are nicely weighted (not too heavy) and all one piece. The four main knives you will need are:

❖ 20cm cook's knife
❖ Paring knife (8, 9 or 10cm)
❖ 14cm vegetable knife
❖ 22cm bread knife (serrated)

A knife sharpener is also worth having to maintain a sharp edge on your knives. I have a ceramic water sharpener.

2. CHOPPING BOARDS

Buy the largest you can find. I like to use a polypropylene one for vegetables (especially onion and garlic) and keep my wooden boards for bread and sweet things. Always place a damp cloth or damp paper towel under your board to stop it from moving when you are chopping.

3. FRY PANS

You need one decent large fry pan for sautéing and pan frying. Decide on size. I recommend one between 20–30cm. Types available include: stainless steel, cast-iron (very heavy), enamel, and copper. Many come with non-stick coating but make sure it is non-toxic (impervious) as some non-stick fry pans, such as those with Teflon, can release toxins.

4. SAUTE PAN OR CASSEROLE DISH

These are perfect for curries, casseroles and chilli. Look for a thick, heavy base. It is definitely worth investing in one that is well made, for example, Le Creuset, Chasseur or Scan Pan, because you will have it for years. We have both a Chasseur pot and a Scan Pan Commercial Grade Sauté Pan with glass lid.

5. SOUP POT

A large soup pot is really handy for making large batches of soup that you can then portion out and freeze.

6. PRESSURE COOKER/SLOW COOKER

A sealed pressure cooker works by using pressure to raise the temperature of water and steam above the normal boiling point of 100°C. Food therefore cooks faster whilst retaining its nutrients.

If you are cooking your own dried beans and chickpeas, a pressure cooker can save a LOT of time. Beans that take almost an hour on the stove can take as little as 3 minutes in the pressure cooker. Chickpeas take only 18 minutes. I love to cook batches of beans in my pressure cooker, then portion them up in the same size you get in a tin, which is roughly 1⅓ to 1½ cups and freeze them. Pressure cookers can also be used to make soup, casseroles, curries, chillies and other similar dishes in a hurry.

A note on slow cookers: Some people prefer to use a slow cooker than a pressure cooker, which is another great way to simplify food prep. Pop dinner in your slow cooker before work and let it simmer away so it is ready to eat when you arrive home. These are also a very handy tool, so choose whatever works best for you. Some of my friends have both cookers!

7. WOK

A wok is fabulous if you like to make stir-fries, which are such a quick and easy meal and a terrific and tasty way to eat lots of vegetables. The best thing about them is that you get to toss the veggies around with great gusto, without them landing all over your stove! My favourite way to cook mushrooms is in a wok as they come out golden brown. They can also be used for fried rice style dishes and noodle dishes. The best place to purchase a wok is an Asian grocery store. Get a moderately weighted one as thicker woks will distribute the heat more evenly. Make sure to season it properly.

8. COLANDER

You will need two—a large one for draining pasta, potatoes and when washing veggies especially kale, silver beet (chard) and spinach, and a fine mesh one for draining grains like quinoa, rice, or when washing herbs.

9. MIXING BOWLS

I prefer to use stainless steel ones as they are more durable. It's best to have several different sizes and I like the ones with a lip on the edge as they are easy to hold. Buy a set that stacks neatly inside each other.

10. WOODEN SPOONS

The bigger the better!

11. SILICON SPATULAS/SPOONULAS

Spatulas and spoonulas are great for mixing and scraping out bowls. They are also very easy to wash.

12. MEASURING CUPS AND SPOONS

I prefer stainless steel ones to the usual plastic ones.

You need a cup set with each of the sizes ¼, ⅓, ½, and 1 cup (250 ml).

When buying your spoon set, be aware that in Australia 1 tablespoon = 4 teaspoons = 20 ml. Many sets have the American size, which is 15 ml!

13. GLASS STORAGE CONTAINERS

Pyrex is my favourite. Choose ones with a glass base and plastic lid. Can go from freezer to oven (remove lid first of course!). Don't heat food in the microwave with the lid on. Take it off and use kitchen paper towel to cover while heating instead.

14. VEGETABLE PEELER

If your fruit and veggies are mainly organic, you don't want to use this often! Interestingly, cheaper peelers are often the best.

15. CAN OPENER

You can get fancy ones that take the whole lid off, which I really like, through to super-cheap ones that usually do the job. Whichever one you decide on, make sure to keep it clean.

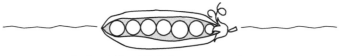

KITCHEN TOOLS

Here is a list of my favourite kitchen tools. Of course, you don't need these, but they are really nice to have. They do make life easier as they make kitchen prep a lot faster and more enjoyable!

1. FOOD PROCESSOR

Really handy for chopping and mixing, especially when making veggie burgers. Some people use blenders but I find food processors more versatile as they can chop, blend, purée, mix and knead, and many come with attachments you can use to grate or slice. Blenders are great for liquidising things like juices and smoothies, but you can also make smoothies in a food processor.

HOW TO SELECT A FOOD PROCESSOR:

❖ Price—obviously it needs to suit your budget
❖ Size of bowl—decide on which size suits your needs best

❖ Attachments—which would you use? They often come with all sorts of attachments, many of which you will never use!
❖ Size of the motor—usually the bigger and stronger the motor, the more expensive, but will be more robust and more likely to last longer.

Depending on the volume you are producing, you may be able to get away with a stick blender, which is great to blend soups and smoothies. Many come with handy attachments like small bowls that are the perfect size for puréeing beans or making pesto, small batches of dip and curry pastes.

2. MICROPLANES

I love these fancy graters! Microplanes come in three sizes—fine, coarse and extra coarse. I use my fine one the most. Great for lemon zest, garlic, turmeric, ginger, fresh nutmeg.

3. STAINLESS STEEL JUICER

I prefer a stainless steel one as it is sharper and sturdy. It comes with a bowl to catch the juice and is very easy to clean, especially if you wash it soon after use.

4. GARLIC PRESS

Usually the sturdier they are, the more expensive. It will however last you for years. Choose an aluminium or steel one. Avoid ones with a plastic hinge and press because these are more fragile. Wash soon after using as garlic tends to stick as it dries.

I have a Zyliss one that is more than 20 years old and still going strong!

5. KITCHEN SCALES

I have a set of slim-line scales as they are easy to store. I find it much easier to weigh many ingredients straight into a bowl, especially sticky ingredients like oil and maple syrup, and there is less washing up. Also weighing ingredients is more accurate than measuring in cups and spoons, but this is usually only important when baking.

6. MANDOLIN

Mandolins are fabulous to slice, shred and julienne lots of veggies in a small amount of time and in uniform size. ALWAYS USE THE HAT to protect your hands! Without the hat, the mandolin is the most lethal kitchen tool.

7. ELECTRIC GRATER (IF YOU DON'T HAVE A FOOD PROCESSOR)

I have a fabulous electric grater which I use all the time to grate carrot and beetroot for salads, and other veggies like zucchini, potato, sweet potato and pumpkin for burgers and fritters.

8. SPIRALISER

A great way to encourage you to eat more veggies, and kids LOVE them. Often you can find lots of helpers in your kitchen when you have one of these! Use a spiraliser to make 'noodles' from veggies such as zucchini, cucumber, sweet potato, regular potato, carrot, pumpkin and beetroot. You can also use a spiraliser to shred onion and cabbage. And you can even 'spiralise' fruit.

COOKING TIPS

SETTING YOURSELF UP FOR SUCCESS

Given the time it takes to prepare meals, one of the best things you can do is batch cook or cook once but make two or more meals from your effort. For example, Bolognese sauce can be used as a topping for roasted sweet potato, add kidney beans and chilli powder to transform it into chilli, serve on top of corn chips for healthy nachos or make it into a cottage pie by topping it with mash and bake until golden.

Here are some more tips on how to streamline your cooking process:

BEFORE YOU START COOKING:

❖ Clear your bench so you have plenty of space to lay out your ingredients and room to work
❖ Wipe the bench down thoroughly
❖ Read through your recipe so you are familiar with the steps and equipment needed. Get the equipment out, ready to use
❖ Put a wet piece of kitchen paper towel under your chopping board to stop it moving
❖ Gather your ingredients and measure them out
❖ If the oven needs preheating, turn it on so it is ready. If it doesn't need preheating, save energy by turning it on at the last minute.

WHEN FINISHED:

❖ Remember to turn everything off—stoves, oven etc.
❖ Put away ingredients and equipment that you no longer need
❖ Place food or leftovers in containers ready for storage in the fridge or freezer, but make sure the food is cold before doing so
❖ Wash up dirty bowls, pans etc.
❖ Scrub chopping board
❖ Wipe surface down thoroughly
❖ Sweep the floor and clean up anything that may have spilled with kitchen paper towel. Never use the kitchen cloth that you use on the benches to wipe the floor!

Notes

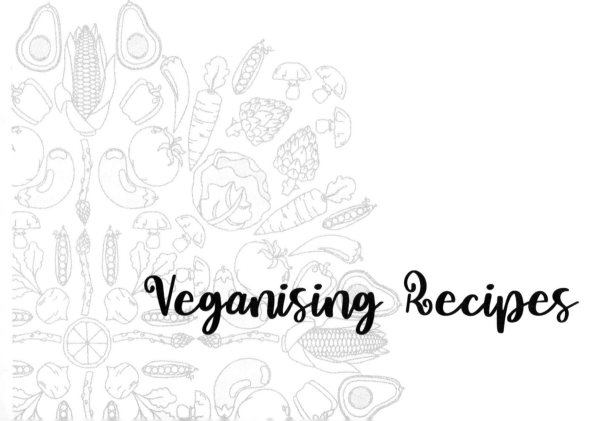

Veganising Recipes

When it comes to making delicious vegan meals and snacks, there are already plenty of vegan recipe books on the market. As an additional option, however it is often quite easy to tweak vegetarian recipes. Of course, some recipes will be easier to adapt than others, plus the more you experiment, the easier it will be to make these changes.

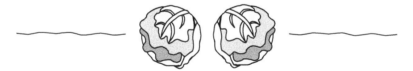

TRY SOME OF THESE EASY SWAPS:

❖ Use cashew or other vegan cheese in place of feta or other dairy-based cheeses.
❖ Sprinkle pasta and other baked goods with nutritional yeast in place of parmesan cheese.
❖ Try linseed egg replacer in veggie burgers (see details on following page), muffins and many cakes.
❖ For ricotta toppings on lasagne, make a white sauce using a plant milk and cornflour or simply blend a small packet each of firm and soft tofu together with a little soymilk. Flavour it by adding nutritional yeast and/or cashew cheese if you like.

BAKING SWAPS

In heavier, fruit-based cakes and muffins that already use an oil for the fat component, use an egg replacer as listed on the following page. My favourite is the linseed egg.

Butter in baked goods can often be replaced with coconut oil but will of course have a slight coconut flavour. Alternatively, you could try half coconut oil and half olive oil. Butter can also be replaced with vegan margarine, but I don't recommend using margarine because it is highly processed. I personally prefer to use less refined products.

Vegan baking and cooking swaps

Non vegan Ingredient	Vegan ingredient	Quantity needed	Where to use swap
Eggs	My favourite option is linseeds + water	1 tablespoon ground linseeds + 3 tablespoons water = 1 egg	Any option can be used in moist baked goods, e.g., muffins, cakes, some biscuits. I prefer to use linseed eggs in veggie burgers
	Bananas	½ banana = 1 egg	
	Apple sauce	¼ cup apple sauce = 1 egg	
	Silken tofu	¼ cup whipped tofu = 1 egg	
	Commercial egg replacers	Refer to instructions on pack	
Milk	Use any nut, seed or grain milk. Commercial brands all vary in flavour and thickness, plus some are sweetened vs unsweetened	1:1	Straight swap
Buttermilk	Add 1 tablespoon of vinegar or lemon juice per 1 cup plant milk and allow to stand for 10 minutes	1:1	Straight swap

Notes

Recipes:
a few Vegan Basics

NUT MILK

Making your own nut milk is quick, easy and much cheaper than buying it. Plus you avoid any additives and can add your own level of sweetening to it if you like. Any nut can be used and sesame seeds can also be incorporated to boost the calcium content.

Nut milk can replace dairy milk in drinks and recipes. It's also delicious flavoured with chocolate, cinnamon, dates, vanilla or even coconut.

INGREDIENTS

- ❖ 1 cup raw nuts of choice (cashew, almond, macadamia etc.)
- ❖ 2–4 cups water, plus extra for soaking

DIRECTIONS

1. Soak the nuts at room temperature overnight, or for a faster version, cover with boiling water and soak until the water has cooled down (approximately 30 minutes to 1 hour)

2. Drain nuts. Place soaked nuts in your food processor or blender. Blend for 30 seconds to 1 minute, until they form a smooth paste. Slowly add 2 cups of water into the blender while it is turned on. Blend well for 1 minute or so until well combined. How long this takes depends on the speed of your blender. Use as is or add extra water depending on how thick you like your milk.

   Many people use a fine mesh sieve to strain the milk to remove any solid particles (nut meal). Alternatively, you can use a cheesecloth or nut bag to strain the milk, as you can squeeze out the last dregs of milk using your hands. I don't bother with this step as I find my nut milk hardly contains any bits. Plus, it doesn't bother me if there are a few little crunchy bits at the bottom of my cup or glass.

3. Storage: I store my nut milk in a glass bottle in the fridge. Fresh nut milk will keep in the fridge for at least 3 days. You can also freeze it. Note that nut milks can naturally separate. This is nothing to worry about, just give them a good stir or shake before use. To sweeten your nut milk: Add 1 to 2 pitted Medjool dates and a dash of pure vanilla essence. Blend.

COCONUT MILK

To make a coconut nut milk (which can be used in cooking): Place 1 cup of shredded coconut or dried coconut flakes in a small bowl and cover with 1 cup of boiling water. Leave to soak until cool. Add this mixture to the nuts and water in Step 2 of the nut milk recipe on the previous page and blend together well.

Sesame seeds can be used to boost calcium content. They are lovely combined with most nuts.

SOUR 'CREAM'

Here are two versions for vegan sour 'cream'. Both are delicious on top of soups, healthy nachos, burritos, burrito bowls, baked regular or sweet potatoes, and possibly certain grainy salads.

SUNFLOWER SEED SOUR 'CREAM'

INGREDIENTS

- ❖ ½ cup raw sunflower seeds
- ❖ ½ cup water
- ❖ 2 tablespoons freshly squeezed lemon juice
- ❖ ¼ teaspoon sea salt
- ❖ ¼ teaspoon onion or garlic powder, optional

DIRECTIONS

1. In a high-powered blender, combine the sunflower seeds, water, lemon juice, and sea salt.
2. Blend on high for 3 to 5 minutes or until completely smooth.
3. Pour into an airtight jar and refrigerate until ready to use.

TOFU SOUR 'CREAM'

INGREDIENTS

- ❖ 300 g soft silken tofu, drained
- ❖ 1 small clove garlic, crushed
- ❖ 2 tablespoons freshly squeezed lemon juice
- ❖ 1 tablespoon extra virgin olive oil
- ❖ ½ teaspoon Dijon mustard

DIRECTIONS

1. Place tofu, garlic, lemon juice, oil and mustard in the bowl of a food processor and process until smooth.
2. Pour into an airtight jar or container and refrigerate until ready to use.

SWEET CASHEW CREAM

Cashew cream is absolutely delicious and very, very versatile. It makes a fabulous topping for fruit salad, pancakes, served alongside fresh berries, stewed fruit or other desserts. Use it as a topping or filling for cupcakes or simply serve alongside a slice of freshly baked cake. Yum!

INGREDIENTS

- ❖ ½ cup raw cashew nuts
- ❖ 2 canned pear halves, drained or 1 ripe fresh, peeled and cored pear
- ❖ ½ teaspoon vanilla essence

DIRECTIONS

1. Place cashews, pear and vanilla in a food processor and purée for several minutes until really smooth.
2. Scrape down the sides of the bowl with a spatula and process again for a few seconds to fully incorporate all ingredients.
3. Serve immediately or store in the fridge for up to 5 days.

LIQUID GOLD DRESSING

Adapted from Becoming vegan: The complete guide to adopting a healthy plant-based diet by Davis and Melina.

A fabulous dressing that can be used to dress up any salad.

1½ tablespoons of this dressing provides 3.5 grams of omega-3 fatty acids, which is almost a day's supply, along with 1.8mcg or 75 percent of your daily vitamin B12 intake if using ¼ cup nutritional yeast in the recipe. This is dependent of course upon how much vitamin B12 is in your nutritional yeast. Nutritional analysis was done using the nutritional yeast mentioned on page 58.

INGREDIENTS

- ❖ ½ cup (125 ml) flaxseed oil
- ❖ ½ cup (125 ml) water
- ❖ ⅓ cup (80 ml) freshly squeezed lemon juice
- ❖ ¼ cup (60 ml) tamari or light soy sauce
- ❖ 1½ tablespoons (30 ml) balsamic vinegar
- ❖ ¼–½ cup (25–50 g) nutritional yeast
- ❖ 2 teaspoon Dijon mustard
- ❖ 1 teaspoon ground cumin
- ❖ ½ teaspoon ground turmeric
- ❖ Black pepper, to taste

DIRECTIONS

1. Place all ingredients in the bowl of a food processor or into a large jug if using a stick blender and blend until smooth.
2. Transfer to a glass jar with a tight-fitting lid.
3. Store in the fridge for up to 2 weeks.
4. Makes approximately 2 cups.

List of Vegan Recipes

Available on healthyhomecafe.com You can find the following vegan recipes along with photos on my website, Healthy Home Café at www.healthyhomecafe.com.

Some recipes may need a small vegan swap (like substituting cheese), but most are already vegan.

BREAKFAST

Banana, Macadamia, Maple Syrup and Cinnamon Granola

Bircher Muesli

Buckwheat Granola

Carrot and Quinoa Seed Loaf

Chia Breakfast Puds

Fig and Hazelnut Toasted Muesli

Mango Chia Breakfast Trifles

Nutty Granola

LUNCHES AND DINNERS

Lighter Meals

3 Minute Bean Burritos

Cannellini Bean and Zucchini Burgers (use egg replacer)

Carrot and Zucchini Croquettes (use egg replacer)

Cauliflower Falafels

Mushroom Lentil and Walnut Tart

Pan-fried Falafels with Lemony Tahini Sauce

Quick Veggie Pakoras

Super-fast Nachos (use vegan cheese)

Salads

Black Beluga Lentils with Rocket, Pumpkin, Beetroot and Avocado

Kale Slaw

Kale, Quinoa, Edamame and Avocado Salad

Marinated Bean Salad

Moroccan Roasted Cauliflower and Chickpea Salad

My Favourite Brown Rice Salad

Nutty Quinoa Salad

Pesto Pasta Salad

Roasted Pumpkin Salad

Spinach and Tahini Slaw

Spinach Green Bean and Walnut Salad

Warm Quinoa Salad with Roasted Cauliflower, Fennel and Pomegranate

Soups

Broccoli and Pea Soup

Broccoli and Red Lentil Soup with Sesame Roasted Kale

Cannellini Bean and Kale Soup

Carrot and Red Lentil Soup with Cashew Cheese, Dukkah and Seedy Soda Bread Rolls

Carrot Leek and White Bean Soup

Carrot Soup with Cashews, Coconut Milk and Coriander

Cauliflower, Red Lentil and Coconut Soup

Creamy Curried Cauliflower and Cashew Soup

Cumin Spiced Lentil and Spinach Soup

French Onion Soup (with an Australian Twist) (replace Gruyere with cashew cheese)

Gazpacho

Green Pea Soup

Minestrone Verde (Spring Minestrone)

Miso Soup with Kale

Moroccan Pumpkin and Chickpea Soup

Mushroom Leek and Barley Soup

Pumpkin Leek and Red Lentil Soup

Quick Minestrone

Red Lentil Soup with Tomatoes and Zucchini

Roasted Carrot Turmeric and Coconut Soup

Roasted Pumpkin Soup with Black Beans and Coriander

Roasted Tomato and Capsicum Soup with Roasted Chickpeas

Spicy Tomato Lentil and Chickpea Soup

Thai Style Pumpkin Soup with Coconut and Red Lentils

Turkish Red Lentil Soup

White Bean, Sweet Paprika and Roasted Capsicum Soup with Crostini

Zucchini Corn and Coriander Soup

Baked Eggplant, Chickpeas and Green Chilli

Black Bean Burrito Bowls

Black Bean Burritos

Black Bean Soft Tacos

Cauliflower Fried Rice

Cauliflower Pizza with Zaatar and Tahini (replace egg with linseed egg)

Eggplant and Chickpea Parmigiana

Eggplant Pumpkin and Chickpea Curry

Eggplant, Dhal and Roti

Fast Fabulous Bean Chilli with Lime and Avocado

Lentil and Cashew Loaf

Lentil Bolognese

Red Lentil, Eggplant and Basil Lasagne (use vegan 'cheese' sauce as topping)

Roasted Pumpkin and Peanut Curry

Stir Fried Veggies with Soy and Basil Tofu

SNACKS
Savoury Snacks

Edamame Hummus

Hummus

Thai Lime and Chilli Hummus

Seedy Crackers

Sweet Snacks and Baking

Anzac Biscuits with Macadamia Nuts

Apple Walnut and Oat Bars

Apricot, Date, Macadamia and Ginger Biscuits

Banana Date and Walnut Bread

Caramel or Chocolate Bliss (Energy) Balls

Chocolate Cake with Apple and Banana

Chocolate Raspberry Brownies

Chocolate, Pecan and Raisin Biscuits

Crunchy Quinoa Muesli Bars

Energy Balls

Ginger Cake

Ginger Nut Biscuits

Healthy Christmas Cake

Jam-filled Oat Bran Muffins

Lemon Bars

Lime Bites

Muesli Bars

No-Bake Seedy Chocolate Energy Bars

Nut Bars

Peanut Butter Chickpea Energy Balls

Raspberry Chia Jam Drop Cookies (Raw)

Raspberry Oat Bars

Seedy Apricot and Tahini Balls (Nut Free)

Sesame and Nut Protein Bars

Super Seedy Crunchy Cookies

Tahini Biscuits

DESSERTS

Banana Caramel Ice Cream

Banana Coconut Ice Cream

Berry Gelato

Chocolate Chia Puddings

Chocolate Mousse Tart with Raspberry Coulis

Coconut and Vanilla Bean Panna Cotta

Mango Coconut Ice Cream

Strawberry Santas

APPENDIX

COMMON ANIMAL-DERIVED INGREDIENTS

Carmine/Cochineal/Carminic Acid, also known as Crimson Lake, Natural Red 4 or E120, is red pigment from crushed female cochineal insects who have bright red shells. Often used as a red food colouring.

Casein and similar-sounding substances are milk proteins which are often used in soy cheeses.

Collagen and keratin are rendered proteins from slaughtered animals.

Gelatine is derived from the skin, bones, tendons or ligaments of animals. Often used in lollies, marshmallows, jelly and as a preservative.

Isinglass is a form of gelatine from fish used in the clarification or 'clearing' of some wines.

Lactose is a sugar extracted from milk.

Lanolin, also known as wool fat, comes from the oil glands of sheep. Widely used in cosmetics.

Lard and tallow are both animal fat. Often used in baked goods, frozen French fries and some refried beans.

Rennet is an enzyme from calves' stomachs used in cheese-making and to make junket (custard).

Vitamin D can come from fish liver oil and other animal products but can also come from plant sources. Vitamin D2 is typically vegan, however vitamin D3 may come from animal sources.

Whey is a milk-based by-product of cheese-making and is often used as a protein boost in some processed foods, such as cakes, biscuits and breads, and in protein powders. Whey can also be soy-based.

Visit Peta (https://www.peta.org/) for a more comprehensive list.

GLOSSARY

CHOLESTEROL

Cholesterol is a fat used in the structure of every cell in your body. In fact the body produces around 800 mg of cholesterol a day as it is used for many other important processes as well. Cholesterol is part of scar tissue that forms to heal a cut or wound, is part of the myelin sheath that coats the nerve fibres in the brain, is the backbone for important hormones and vitamin D and is a component of bile which helps with fat digestion in the gut.

Cholesterol is present in animal foods such as eggs, seafood and offal. There is no cholesterol in plant foods. Your body also converts saturated fat from your intake into cholesterol.

1. LDL cholesterol

LDL or low-density lipoproteins are cholesterol carriers in your body. They attach to cholesterol in the liver and transport it throughout the body to sites where it can be used and also where it can be stored. LDL cholesterol is often called 'bad' as elevated levels are associated with an increased risk of cardiovascular disease.

2. HDL cholesterol

HDL or high-density lipoproteins are cholesterol carriers that help to remove cholesterol from deposits in arteries, returning it to the liver for removal from your body. It is referred to as 'good' cholesterol as high levels are associated with a reduced risk of cardiovascular disease whereas low levels are associated with an increased risk.

TRIGLYCERIDES

Triglycerides are another type of fat in your blood. They are the body's main vehicle for transporting fat to cells for use in metabolic processes. An elevated level of triglycerides is associated with an increased risk of cardiovascular disease.

TRANS FATS

Trans fats are created when vegetable oil is hydrogenated or partially hydrogenated, a process that converts liquid oils into hard, stable fats with a longer shelf life and a high melting point which is desirable for deep frying. Trans fats have been linked with dramatically increasing heart disease risk. Foods that contain trans fats include some margarines, shortening, crackers, biscuits, chips, snack foods and deep-fried foods. Thankfully many of these foods contain egg or dairy, so are not vegan.

REFERENCES

1. Craig, W. J. & Mangels, A. R. (2009). Position of the American Dietetic Association: Vegetarian diets. Journal of the American Dietetic Association, 109, 1266–1282

2. Davis, B. & Melina, V. (2000). Becoming vegan: The complete guide to adopting a healthy plant-based diet. Book Publishing Company

3. Saxelby, C. (2018). Complete food and nutrition companion (2nd ed.). Hardie Grant Books

4. Whitney, E & Rolfes, S (2002). Understanding Nutrition (9th ed.). Wadsworth Publishing

5. Marsh, K., Munn, E. and Baines, S. (2019). Protein and vegetarian diets. [online] Mja.com.au. Available at: https://www.mja.com.au/journal/2013/199/4/protein-and-vegetarian-diets [Accessed 22 Jan. 2019].

6. Magee PJ, Rowland I. Soy products in the management of breast cancer. Curr Opin Clin Nutr Metab Care. 2012;15:586-591.

7. Callaway, J. (2019). Hempseed as a nutritional resource: An overview. [online] Finola.fi. Available at: http://finola.fi/wp-content/uploads/2017/10/Hempseed-Nutrition.pdf [Accessed 22 Jan. 2019].

8. The 19 best prebiotic foods suitable for vegans. [online] Medical News Today. Available at: https://www.medicalnewstoday.com/articles/323214.php [Accessed 22 Jan. 2019].

9. Chalker-Scott L. Environmental significance of anthocyanins in plant stress responses. Photochem Photobiol. 1999;70(1):1-9.

10. De Alzaa, F., Guillaume, C. & Ravetti, L. (2018). Evaluation of chemical and physical changes in different commercial oils during heating. Acta Scientific Nutritional Health, 2(6), 2–11

11. Callaway, J. (2019). Hempseed as a nutritional resource: An overview. [online] Finola.fi. Available at: http://finola.fi/wp-content/uploads/2017/10/Hempseed-Nutrition.pdf [Accessed 22 Jan. 2019].

12. Kris-Etherton, P. M., Taylor, D. S., Yu-Poth, S., Huth, P., Moriarty, K., Fishell, V., Hargrove, R. L., Zhao, G. & Etherton, T. D. (2000). Polyunsaturated fatty acids in the food chain in the United States. The American Journal of Clinical Nutrition, 71(1), 179S–188S <https://doi.org/10.1093/ajcn/71.1.179S>

13. World Health Organization. (2003). Diet, nutrition and the prevention of chronic diseases. Report of the joint WHO/FAO expert consultation Technical Report Series, No. 916. Geneva: World Health Organization

14. Moslehi-Jenabian S, Pedersen LL, Jespersen L. Beneficial effects of probiotic and food borne yeasts on human health. Nutrients. 2010;2(4):449–473 [online] Available at: https://www.ncbi.nlm.nih.gov/pmc/articles/PMC3257658/ [Accessed 23 Jan. 2019].

15. Riebl, S. K. & Davy, B. M. (2013). The hydration equation: Update on water balance and cognitive performance. ACSM's Health & Fitness Journal, 17(6), 21–28

16. Nrv.gov.au. (2019). Nutrients | Nutrient Reference Values. [online] Available at: https://www.nrv.gov.au/nutrients [Accessed 22 Jan. 2019].

17. FoodWorks Version 8 by Xyris Software

ABOUT CAROLINE TRICKEY

APD, B Sc, Nutr and Dietetics Monash University

Caroline Trickey is a qualified dietitian and nutritionist who works in private practice and runs a cooking school and website called Healthy Home Café.

The cooking school is designed to show people how to cook delicious, nutritious food quickly and easily. During the classes, Caroline teaches how food can boost your energy, reduce inflammation (inflammation can encourage weight gain, heart disease, cancer, and worsen symptoms from auto-immune conditions) and get more plant-based foods into your intake, a very healthy thing to do!

In a past life, Caroline ran a successful café and catering business. She has a true love and passion for cooking and wants to show people that food is there to nourish us, for enjoyment and pleasure.

Caroline believes in a healthy balance and avoids diets and shaming foods (i.e. she enjoys all food and bakes a mean cake!). Rather she has a more sensible, practical and balanced approach—one that really works long term!

You can access more than 300 of her delicious recipes and find out more about her cooking classes on her website: www.healthyhomecafe.com

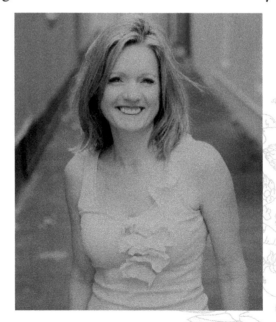

INDEX

Veganism is a way of living which seeks to exclude, as far as is possible and practicable, all forms of exploitation of, and cruelty to, animals for food, clothing or any other purpose.

The Vegan Society 1944

Veganism is the practice of abstaining from the use of animal products, particularly in diet, and an associated philosophy that rejects the commodity status of animals.

A follower of the diet or the philosophy is known as a vegan.

En.wikipedia.org. 2019

Milton Keynes UK
Ingram Content Group UK Ltd.
UKHW050908071223
433828UK00009B/524